The Affordable Anti-Inflammatory Meals

On a Budget Recipes for your Daily Meals

Thomas Jollif

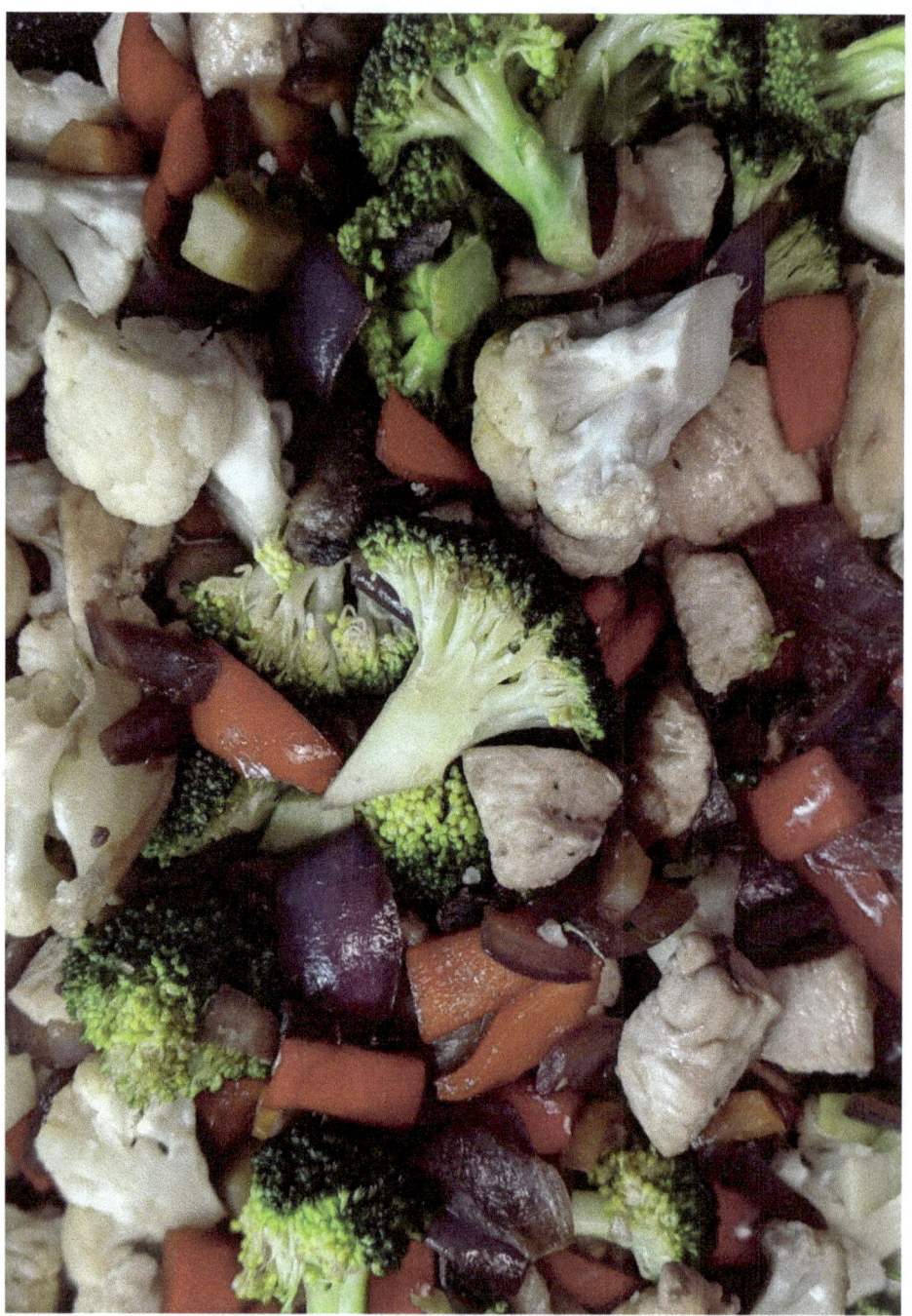

© copyright 2021 – all rights reserved.

the content contained within this book may not be reproduced, duplicated or transmitted without direct written permission from the author or the publisher.

under no circumstances will any blame or legal responsibility be held against the publisher, or author, for any damages, reparation, or monetary loss due to the information contained within this book. either directly or indirectly.

legal notice:

this book is copyright protected. this book is only for personal use. you cannot amend, distribute, sell, use, quote or paraphrase any part, or the content within this book, without the consent of the author or publisher.

disclaimer notice:

please note the information contained within this document is for educational and entertainment purposes only. all effort has been executed to present accurate, up to date, and reliable, complete information. no warranties of any kind are declared or implied. readers acknowledge that the author is not engaging in the rendering of legal, financial, medical or professional advice. the content within this book has been derived from various sources. please consult a licensed professional before attempting any techniques outlined in this book.

by reading this document, the reader agrees that under no circumstances is the author responsible for any losses, direct or indirect, which are incurred as a result of the use of information contained within this document, including, but not limited to, — errors, omissions, or inaccuracies.

Table of Contents

BREAKFASTS 7
- SPINACH MUSHROOM OMELET 7
- STRAWBERRIES AND CREAM TRIFLE 9
- STRAWBERRY YOGURT TREAT 11
- STRAWBERRY-OAT-CHOCOLATE CHIP MUFFINS 13
- SUN-DRIED TOMATO GARLIC BRUSCHETTA 16
- SWEET ONION AND EGG PIE 18
- SWEETENED BROWN RICE 20
- SWISS CHARD AND SPINACH WITH 21
- EGG 21
- TOMATO AND AVOCADO OMELET 23
- TOMATO OMELET 25

SMOOTHIES AND DRINKS 27
- TRIPLE FRUIT SMOOTHIE 27
- TROPICAL MANGO COCONUT SMOOTHIE 29
- TROPICAL PINEAPPLE KIWI SMOOTHIE 31
- TURMERIC AND GINGER TONIC 32
- TURMERIC DELIGHT 35
- TURMERIC HOT CHOCOLATE 36
- TURMERIC TEA 38
- VANILLA AVOCADO SMOOTHIE 40

SIDES 42
- SPICY ROASTED BRUSSELS SPROUTS 42
- SPICY WASABI MAYONNAISE 44

    STIR-FRIED ALMOND AND SPINACH 45

    STIR-FRIED FARROS 47

SAUCES AND DRESSINGS 49

    STRAWBERRY POPPY SEED DRESSING 49

    TAHINI DIP 51

SNACKS 53

    ROASTED GARLIC CHICKPEAS 53

    SALMON & AVOCADO TOAST 55

    SALT & VINEGAR KALE CRISPS 57

    SOFT FLOURLESS COOKIES 59

    SPICED NUTS 61

    SPICY BEAN DIP 63

    SPICY ROASTED CHICKPEAS 65

SOUPS AND STEWS 67

    SPICY CABBAGE TURMERIC COCONUT SOUP 67

    SPICY LIME-CHICKEN "TORTILLA-LESS" SOUP 69

    SPICY RAMEN NOODLES 72

    SPICY SEAFOOD STEW 74

    SWEET POTATO AND BLACK BEAN CHILI 77

    SWEET POTATO AND CORN SOUP 79

    TEX-MEX CHICKEN SOUP 82

    THAI CHICKEN NOODLE SOUP 84

    THAI WINTER VEGETABLE SOUP 86

DESSERTS 88

    SPICED TEA PUDDING 88

    SPICY POPPER MUG CAKE 90

STRAWBERRY GRANITA 93
STRAWBERRY ICE CREAM 95
STRAWBERRY ORANGE SORBET 97
STRAWBERRY SHORTCAKE.. 99
STRAWBERRY SOUFFLÉ *101*
SWEET ALMOND AND COCONUT FAT BOMBS *103*
THE MOST ELEGANT PARSLEY SOUFFLÉ EVER *105*

BREAKFASTS

Spinach Mushroom Omelet

Time To Prepare: three minutes
Time to Cook: fifteen minutes
Yield: Servings 2

Ingredients:

- ¼ Red onion, diced
- 1 ½ cup Spinach, fresh, chopped
- 1 Green onion, diced
- 1 oz. Feta cheese
- 2 tbsp. Olive oil,
- 3 Eggs
- 5 Mushrooms, button, cut

Directions:

1. Sauté the mushrooms, onions, and spinach for 3 minutes in one tablespoon of olive oil and set aside.
2. Beat the eggs thoroughly and cook them in the other tablespoon of olive oil for three to four minutes until edges start to brown. Drizzle all the other ingredients

onto half of the omelet and fold the other half over the sautéed ingredients. Cook for a minute on each side.

Nutritional Info: Calories 337 ‖ 25 grams Fat ‖ 22 grams Protein ‖ 5.4 grams carbs ‖ 1.3 grams sugar ‖ 1 gram fiber

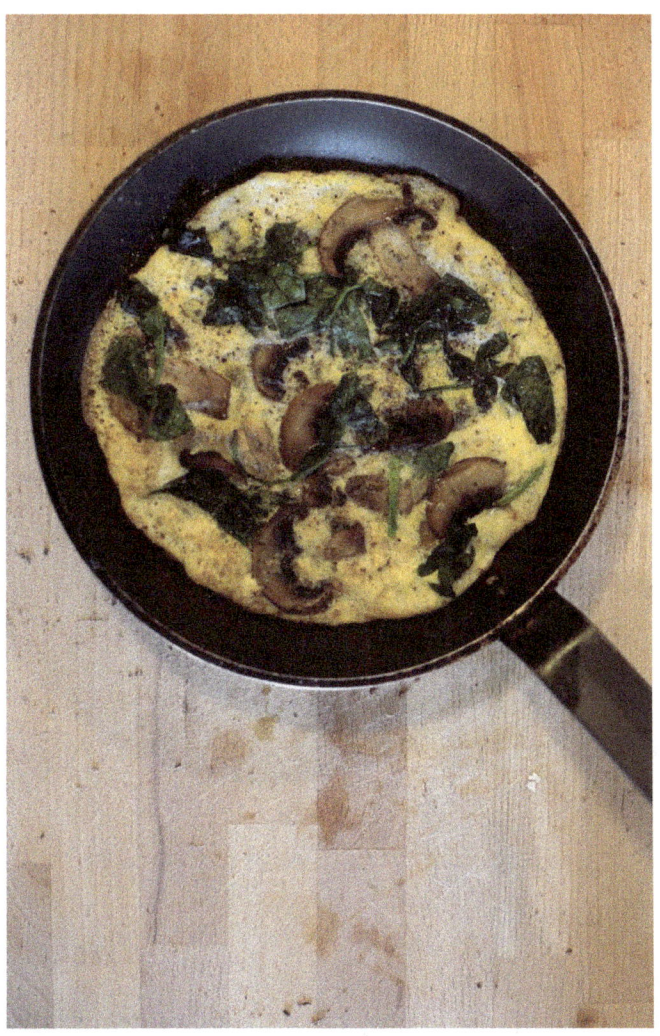

Strawberries and Cream Trifle

Time To Prepare: 10 Minutes
Time to Cook: 45 Minutes
Yield: Servings 12

Ingredients:

- 1 ½ cups condensed milk
- 1 angel food cake, cubed
- 12 ounces frozen whipped cream, thawed
- 3 pints fresh strawberries, hulled and cut
- 6 ounces packaged cream cheese, softened

Directions:

1. In a container, put together the cream cheese, sweetened condensed milk, and whip in until the desired smoothness is achieved.
2. In a trifle container, place a layer of angel food cake cubes. Put in a layer of strawberries and cream on top. Repeat the layers.
3. Bring it in your fridge to cool for minimum thirty-five minutes.

Nutritional Info: Calories: 378 ‖ Fat: 17g ‖ Carbohydrates: 51g ‖ Protein: 7g

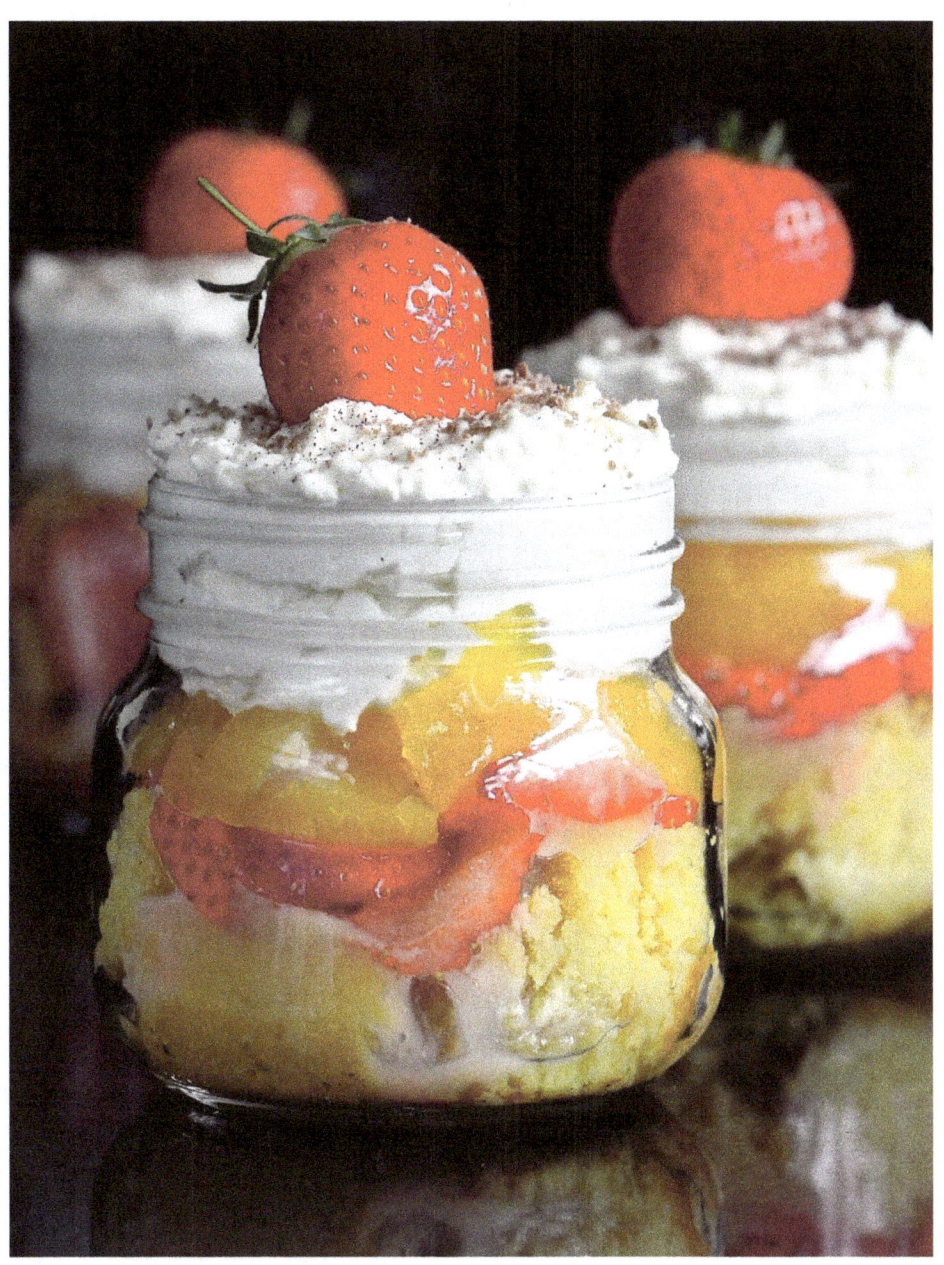

Strawberry Yogurt treat

Time To Prepare: ten minutes
Time to Cook: 0 minutes
Yield: Servings 2

Ingredients:

- 1 cup cut strawberries
- 4 cups 0% Fat plain yogurt
- 4 tbsp. honey
- 8 tbsp. of flax meal
- 8 tbsp. walnuts (chopped)

Directions:

1. Distribute 2 cups of the yogurt into your serving bowls. Neatly layer the flax meal and the walnut in the center.
2. Put in a sprinkle of half of the honey before covering with the final layer of yogurt. Put in the honey on top of the yogurt to put in color when you serve.

Nutritional Info: Calories: 733 kcal ‖ Protein: 38.42 g ‖ Fat: 30.57 g ‖ Carbohydrates: 83.44 g

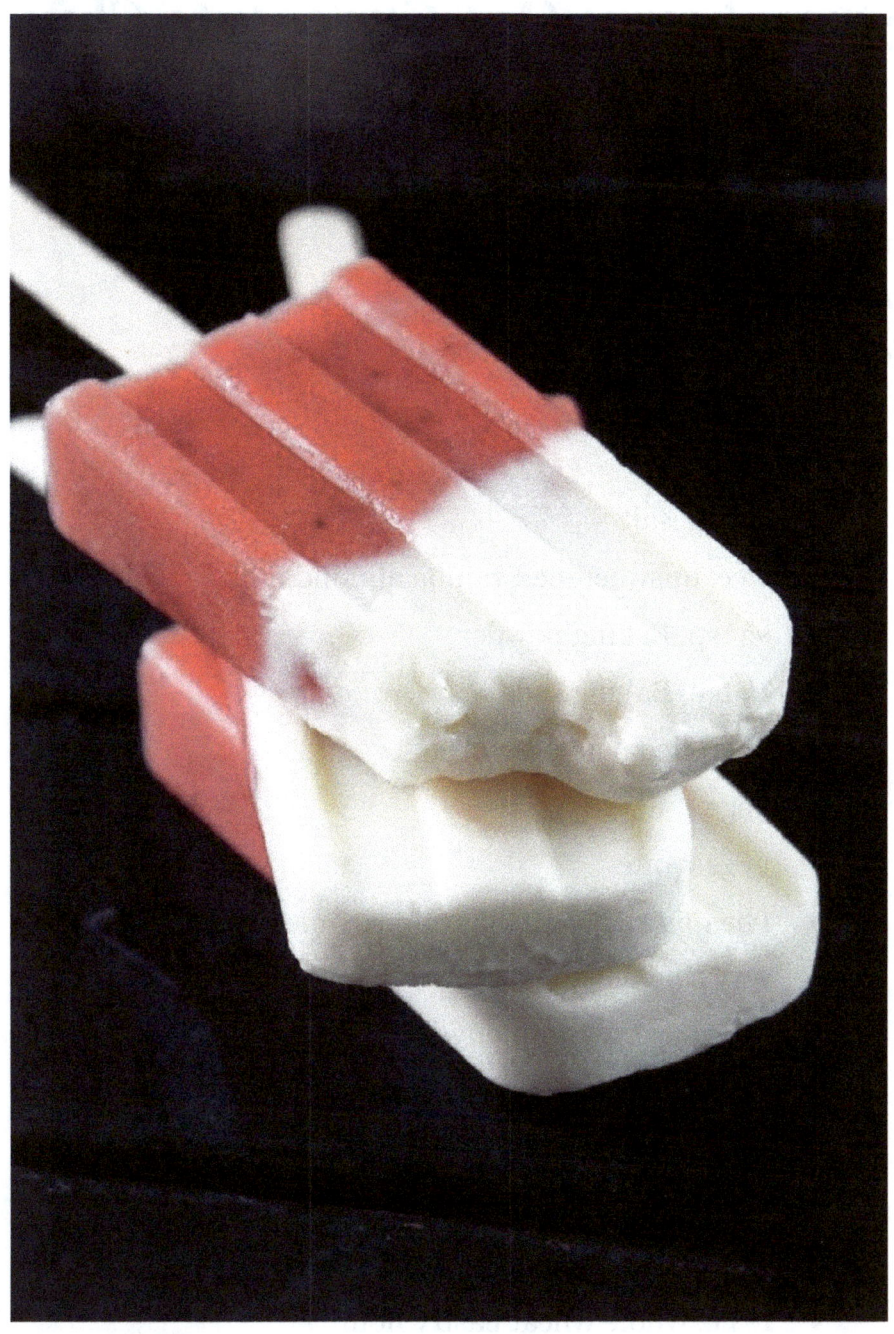

Strawberry-Oat-Chocolate Chip Muffins

Time To Prepare: ten minutes
Time to Cook: 23 minutes
Yield: Servings 12

Ingredients:

- ¼ tsp. salt
- ½ c. unsweetened vanilla almond milk
- ½ tsp. Baking powder
- ¾ tsp. Baking soda
- 1 c. rolled oats
- 1 egg
- 1 egg white
- 1 heaping cup bananas (approximately two to three big very ripe bananas)
- 1 tbsp. extra virgin olive oil
- 1 tbsp. honey or agave nectar
- 1 tsp. vanilla
- 1/3 c. mini chocolate chips
- 1/3 c. nonfat plain Greek yogurt
- 1¼ c. whole wheat pastry flour

- 12 thin slices of strawberries (about 3-4 strawberries) for decoration, if you wish
- 2/3 c. diced strawberries

Directions:

1. Set the oven to 350°F and mildly grease a standard 12-cup muffin pan or grease with paper liners. In a large-sized mixing container, mix flour, oats, baking powder, baking soda, and salt. Stir to blend. Set aside the 2 tbsp. of the mixture.
2. In a different huge mixing container, mix together the mashed banana, olive oil, honey, and vanilla. After this, beat in the egg and egg white and beat until blended. Now put in in Greek yogurt and almond milk and beat using an electric mixer on low until the desired smoothness is achieved.
3. Slowly put wet ingredients to dry ingredients and blend until just blended, but do not over mix the batter as it will make the muffins firm.
4. Fill each muffin cup 2/3 full of batter. Lightly tap the pan on the counter to even out the batter. Put a thin slice of strawberry onto each muffin, if you wish. Place the pan in your oven, then cook for eighteen to 23 minutes, up to a toothpick place in the center of the muffins, and comes out clean. Remove from the oven

and allow it to sit for five to ten minutes in the pan before placing on a cooling rack.

Nutritional Info: Calories: 91 kcal ‖ Protein: 4.02 g ‖ Fat: 2.63 g ‖ Carbohydrates: 16.31 g

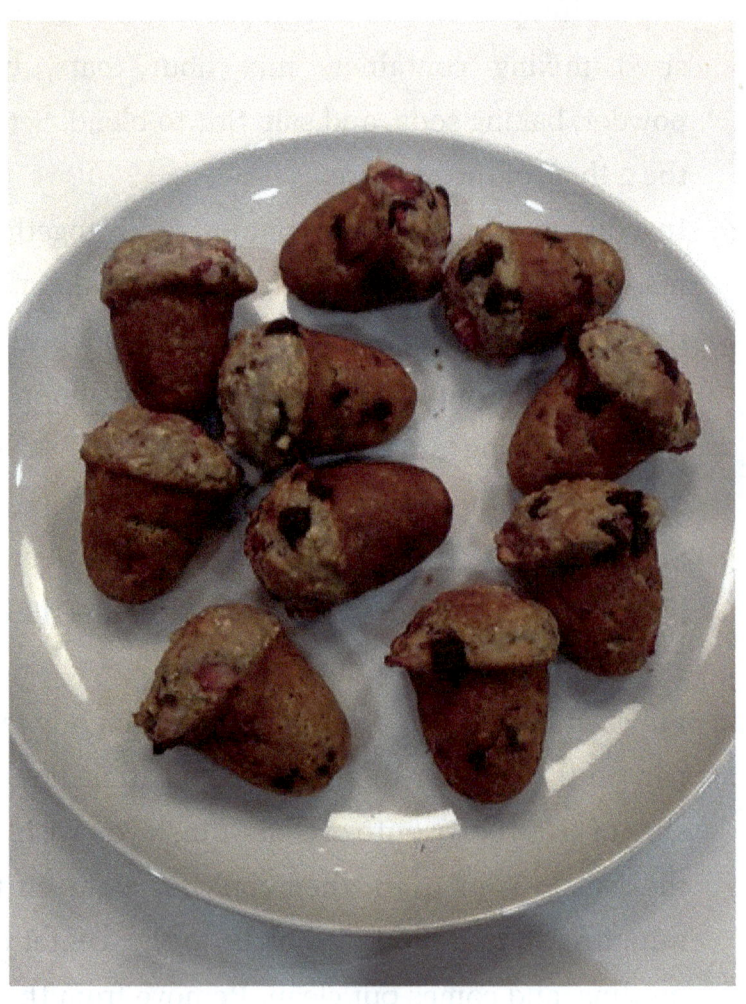

Sun-Dried Tomato Garlic Bruschetta

Time To Prepare: ten minutes
Time to Cook: five minutes
Yield: Servings 6

Ingredients:

- 1 garlic clove, peeled
- 1 tsp. chives, minced
- 1 tsp. olive oil
- 2 slices sourdough bread, toasted
- 2 tsp. sun-dried tomatoes in olive oil, minced

Directions:

1. Vigorously rub garlic clove on 1 side of each of the toasted bread slices
2. Spread equivalent portions of sun-dried tomatoes on the garlic side of bread. Drizzle chives and sprinkle olive oil on top.
3. Pop both slices into oven toaster, and cook until well thoroughly heated.
4. Put bruschetta on a plate. Serve warm.

Nutritional Info: Calories: 149 kcal ‖ Protein: 6.12 g ‖ Fat: 2.99 g ‖ Carbohydrates: 24.39 g

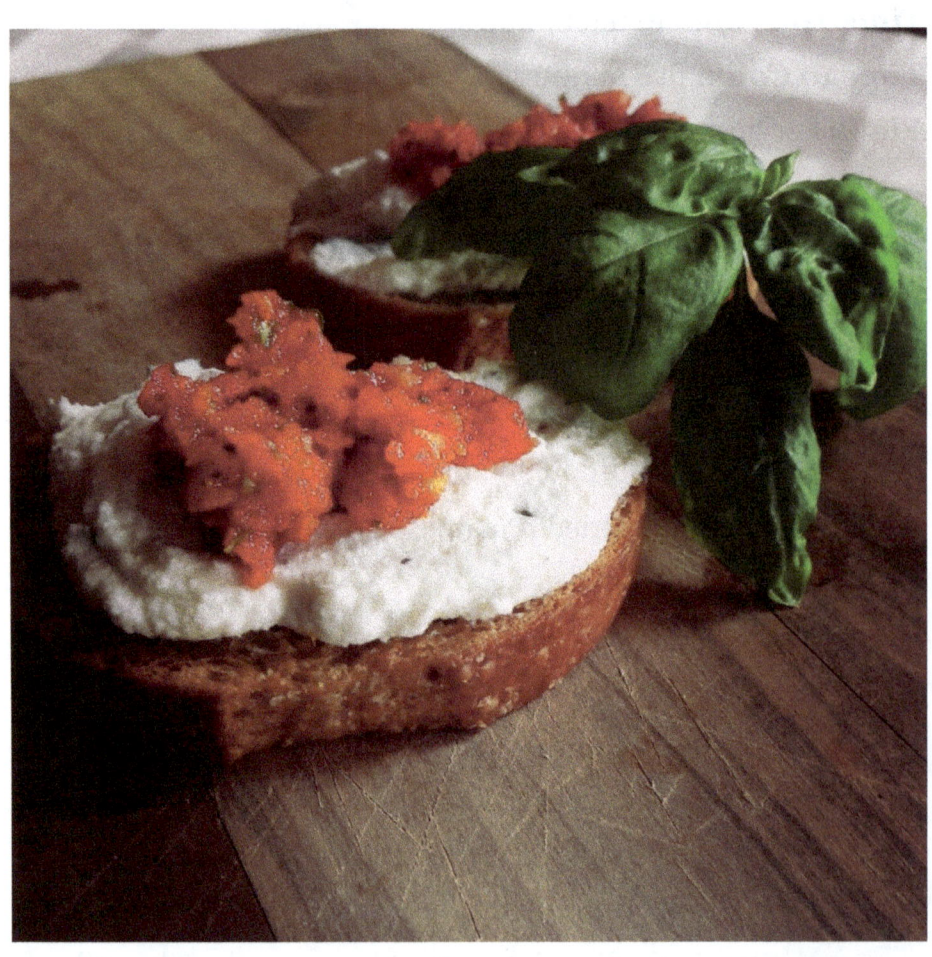

Sweet Onion and Egg Pie

Time To Prepare: 20 Minutes
Time to Cook: 35 Minutes
Yield: Servings 10

Ingredients:

- 1 cup vaporized milk
- 1 tablespoons butter
- 11 frozen deep-dish pie crust
- 2 sweet onions, halved and cut
- 6 eggs
- Salt and pepper to taste

Directions:

1. Preheat your oven 4000F.
2. Melt the butter in a non-stick frying pan. Sauté the onions on moderate to low heat until super soft.
3. Put the onions in a container. Put in in eggs and vaporized milk. Sprinkle with salt and pepper to taste.
4. Pour the egg and onion mixture into the commercial pie crust.
5. Bake using your oven for a little more than half an hour.

Nutritional Info: Calories: 169 ‖ Fat: 7g ‖ Carbohydrates: 21g

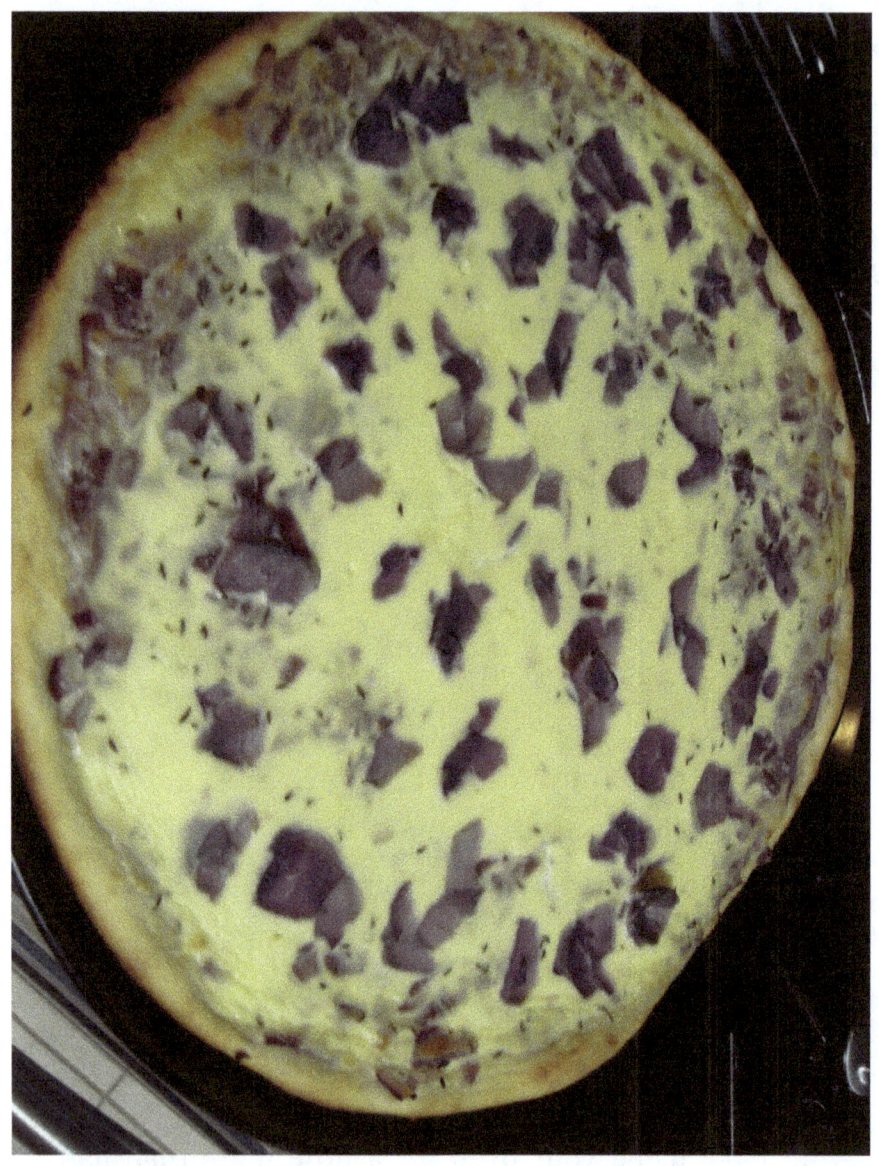

Sweetened Brown Rice

Time To Prepare: ten minutes
Time to Cook: 45-60 minutes
Yield: Servings 8

Ingredients:

- ¼ teaspoon nutmeg
- 1 cup brown rice
- 1 tablespoon honey
- 1½ cups soy milk
- 1½ cups water
- Fresh fruit (not necessary)

Directions:

1. Put all the ingredients excluding the fresh fruit in a medium-size deep cooking pan; put the mixture to a slow simmer then cover using a tight-fitting lid.
2. Simmer for minimum 45-60 minutes, up to the rice is soft and done. Serve in bowls, topped with your favorite fresh fruit.

Nutritional Info: Calories: 155 ‖ Fat: 1.5 g ‖ Protein: 3.5 g ‖ Sodium: 35 mg ‖ Fiber: 1.5 g ‖ Carbohydrates: 13 g

Swiss Chard and Spinach with Egg

Time To Prepare: five minutes
Time to Cook: ten minutes
Yield: Servings 4

Ingredients:

- 1 tsp. olive oil
- 20 pieces spinach leaves
- 20 pieces Swiss chard leaves
- 4 egg whites
- 4 pieces of rice bread
- 4 tbsp. parsley (fresh)
- Sea salt, ground pepper, and dried mint

Directions:

1. Bring to its boiling point 2 cups of water in a pan just below the boiling point. Open an egg, separate the whites from the yolks. Place the whites in a small container. Lower the container towards the heated water, and gently pour the egg into the pan. Do the same with the other eggs. Poach the eggs for about four minutes. Next, gently take the eggs, one by one

and move them into a plate. Do the same with the rest of the 2 eggs.

2. Cut the parsley and sauté the leaves in a pan for about six minutes. Toast the bread while doing this. When finished, make a layer of the sautéed greens and the chopped parsley on top of the toasted rice bread. Place the poached eggs above the bed of greens. Drizzle each serving with ground pepper, sea salt, and dried mint.

Nutritional Info: Calories: 49 kcal ‖ Protein: 5.31 g ‖ Fat: 2.73 g ‖ Carbohydrates: 0.48 g

Tomato and Avocado Omelet

Time To Prepare: five minutes
Time to Cook: five minutes
Yield: Servings 1

Ingredients:

- ¼ avocado, diced
- 1 tablespoon cilantro, chopped
- 2 eggs
- 4 cherry tomatoes, halved
- Pinch of salt
- Squeeze of lime juice

Directions:

1. Put together the avocado, tomatoes, cilantro, lime juice, and salt in a small container, then mix thoroughly and save for later.
2. Warm a moderate-sized nonstick frying pan on moderate heat. Whisk the eggs until frothy and put in to the pan. Move the eggs around gently using a rubber spatula until they start to set.
3. Spread the avocado mixture over half of the omelet. Turn off the heat, and slide the omelet onto a plate as you fold it in half.

4. Serve instantly.

Nutritional Info: Calories: 433 kcal ‖ Protein: 25.55 g ‖ Fat: 32.75 g ‖ Carbohydrates: 10.06 g

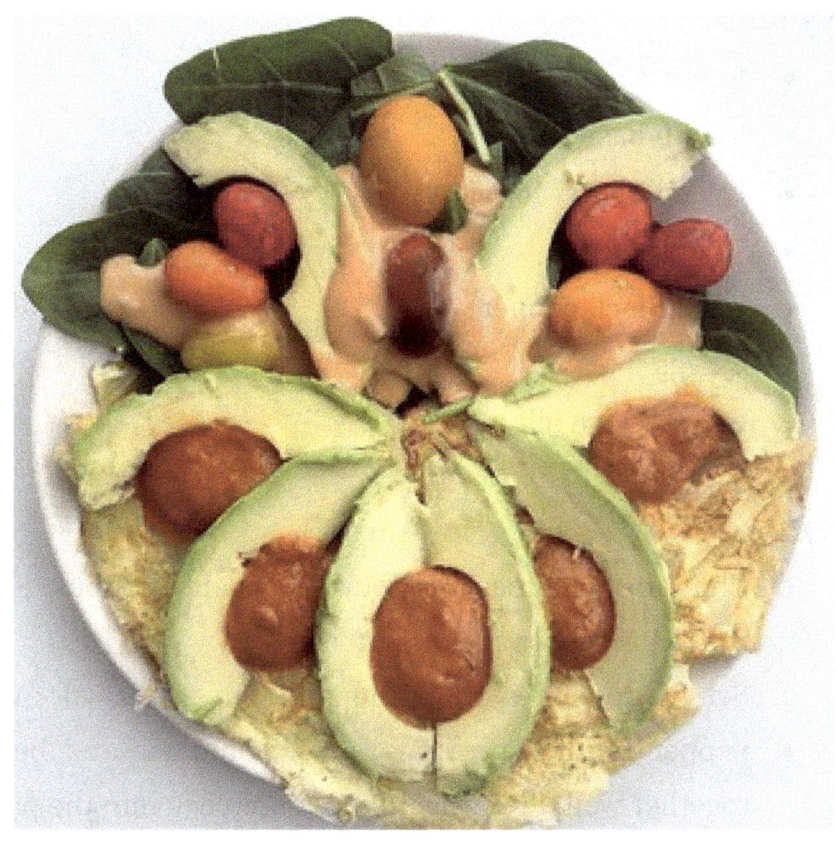

Tomato Omelet

Time To Prepare: two minutes
Time to Cook: 8 minutes
Yield: Servings 1

Ingredients:

- ¼ cup Cheese, any type, shredded
- ½ cup Basil, fresh
- ½ cup Cherry tomatoes
- ½ tsp. Salt
- 1 tsp. Black pepper
- 2 Eggs
- 2 tbsp. Olive oil

Directions:

1. Chop the tomatoes into four equivalent portions. Fry the tomatoes for around three hours.
2. Set the tomatoes off to the side. Put in the salt and pepper to the eggs in a small container and beat together well. Pour the mix of beaten egg into the pan and use a spatula to gently work around the edges under the omelet, letting the eggs fry unmoved for 3 minutes.

3. When just the center third of the egg mix is still runny, put in on the basil, tomatoes, and cheese. Fold over half of the omelet onto the other half. Cook two more minutes before you serve.

Nutritional Info: Calories 342 ∥ 8 grams carbs ∥ 20 grams Protein ∥ 25.3 grams fat

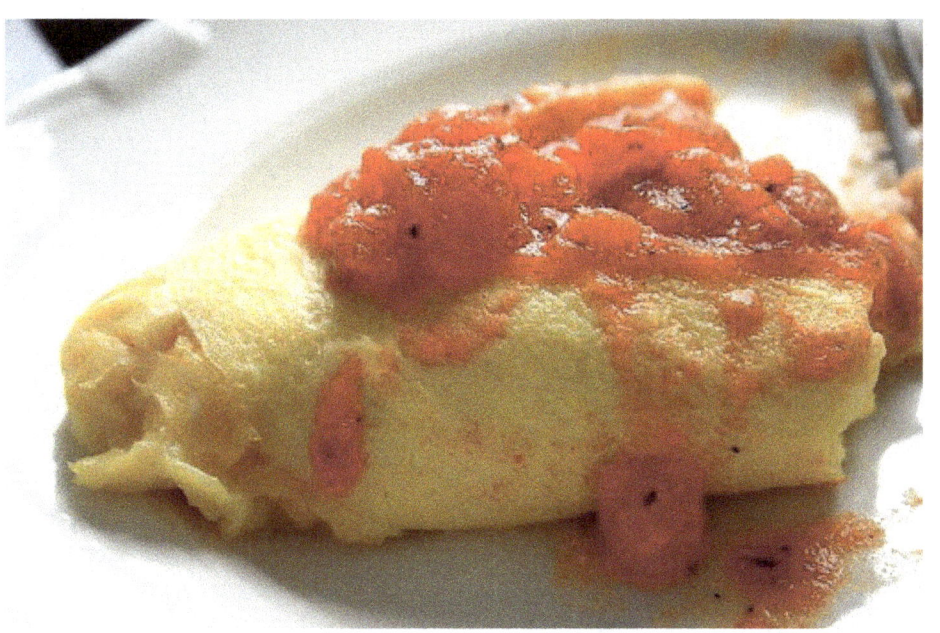

SMOOTHIES AND DRINKS

Triple Fruit Smoothie

Time To Prepare: ten minutes
Time to Cook: 0 minutes
Yield: Servings 1

Ingredients:

- 1 banana, peeled and chopped
- 1 container (8 oz.) peach yogurt
- 1 cup ice cubes
- 1 cup strawberries
- 1 kiwi, cut
- 1/2 cup blueberries
- 1/2 cup orange juice

Directions:

1. Put in everything to a blender jug.
2. Cover the jug firmly.
3. Blend until the desired smoothness is achieved. Serve and enjoy!

Nutritional Info: Calories: 124 ‖ Fat: 0.4 g ‖ Protein: 5.6 g ‖ Carbohydrates: 8 g ‖ Fiber: 2.3 g

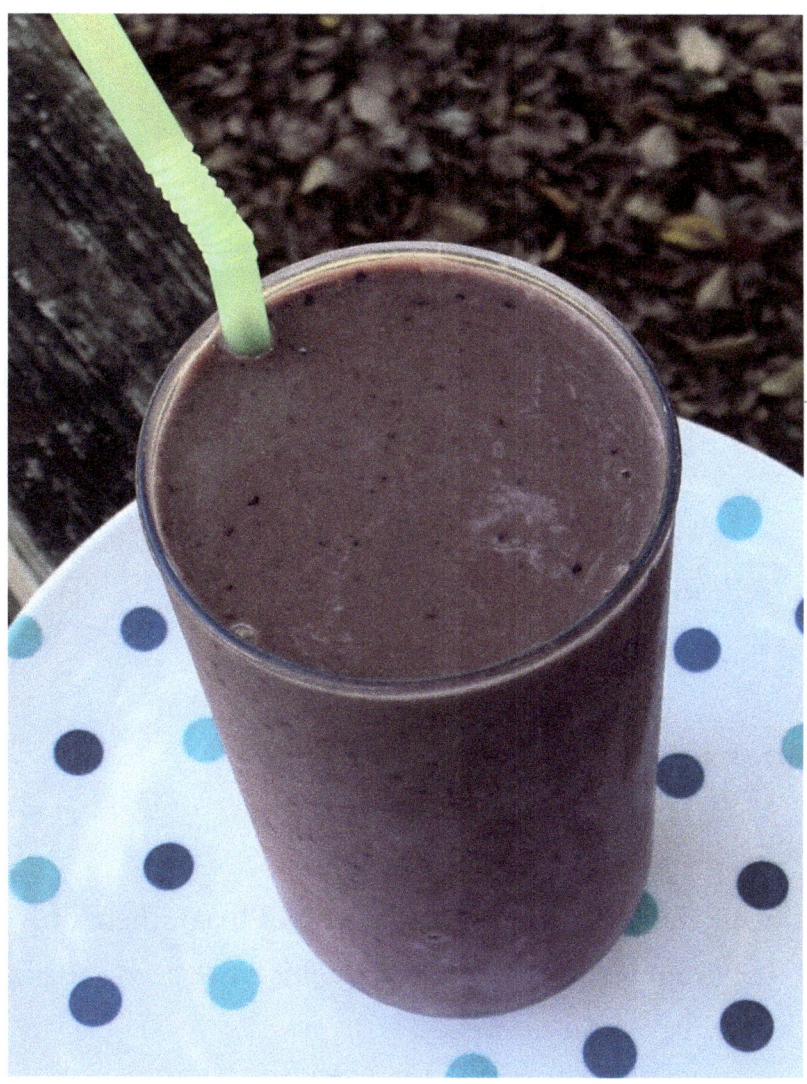

Tropical Mango Coconut Smoothie

Time To Prepare: five minutes
Time to Cook: 0 minutes
Yield: Servings 2

Ingredients:

- ½ cup of canned coconut milk
- ½ cup of fresh orange juice
- 1 ½ cups of frozen mango
- 1 ½ tsp of honey
- 1 medium frozen banana
- 1 tbsp. of fresh lemon juice

Directions:

1. Mix the smoothie ingredients in your high-speed blender.
2. Pulse the ingredients a few times to cut them up.
3. Combine the mixture on the highest speed setting for thirty to 60 seconds.
4. Pour into glasses and serve.

Nutritional Info: Calories: 354 kcal ‖ Protein: 6.7 g ‖ Fat: 18.09 g ‖ Carbohydrates: 47.42 g

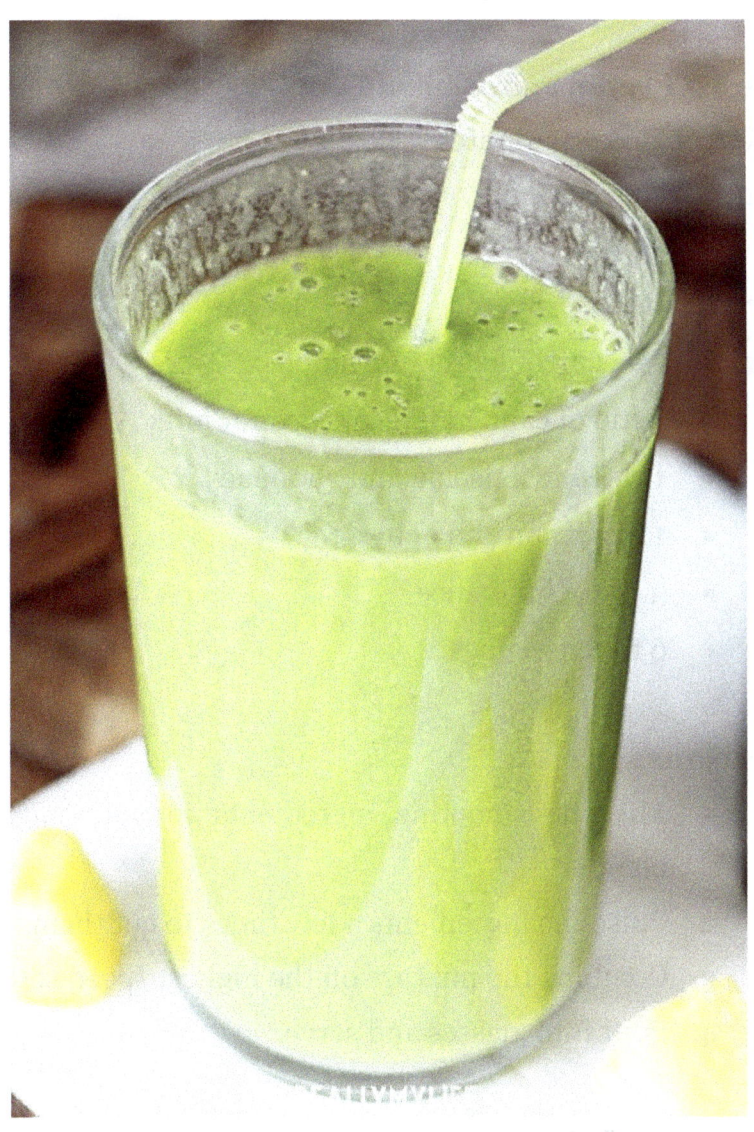

Tropical Pineapple Kiwi Smoothie

Time To Prepare: five minutes
Time to Cook: 0 minutes
Yield: Servings 2

Ingredients:

- 1 ½ cup of frozen pineapple
- 1 cup of canned full-fat coconut milk
- 1 ripe kiwi; peeled and chopped
- 1 tsp of spirulina powder
- 3 tsp of lime juice
- 6 to 8 ice cubes

Directions:

1. Mix the smoothie ingredients in your high-speed blender.
2. Pulse the ingredients a few times to cut them up.
3. Combine the mixture on the highest speed setting.
4. Pour into glasses and serve.

Nutritional Info: Calories: 480 kcal ‖ Protein: 7.38 g ‖ Fat: 31.92 g ‖ Carbohydrates: 48.35 g

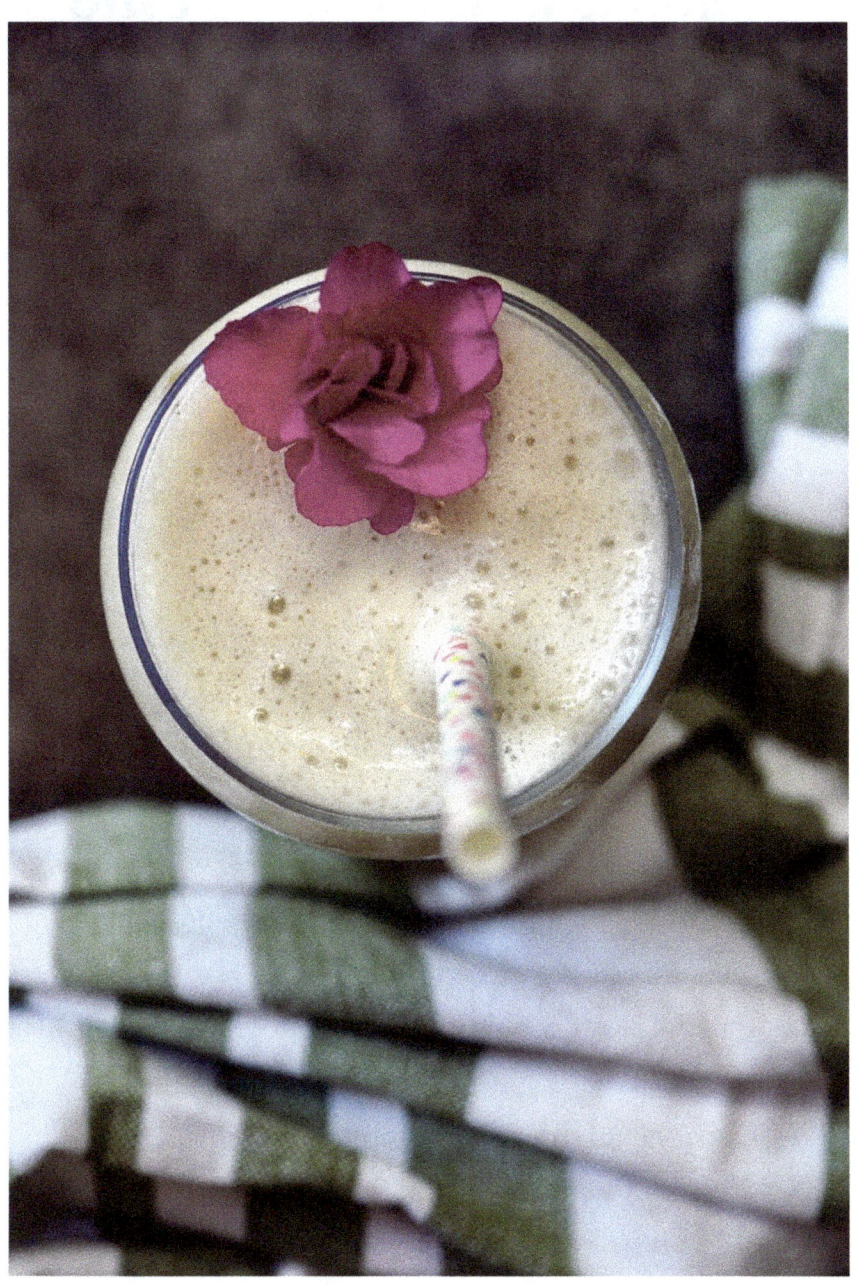

Turmeric and Ginger Tonic

Time To Prepare: five minutes
Time to Cook: ten minutes
Yield: Servings 4

Ingredients:

- 1/8 teaspoon cayenne pepper
- 2 tablespoons grated, fresh ginger
- 2 tablespoons grated, fresh turmeric
- 6 cups water
- Juice of 2 lemons
- Maple syrup or honey to taste
- The rind of 2 lemons, peeled

Directions:

1. Put in water, ginger, turmeric, cayenne pepper, and lemon rind into a deep cooking pan.
2. Put the deep cooking pan on moderate to high heat. (Do not boil)
3. Once the mixture is hot, remove from heat.
4. Strain into 4 mugs. Put in honey and lemon juice and stir.
5. Serve warm.

Nutritional Info: Calories: 48 kcal ‖ Protein: 2.28 g ‖ Fat: 1.81 g ‖ Carbohydrates: 7.03 g

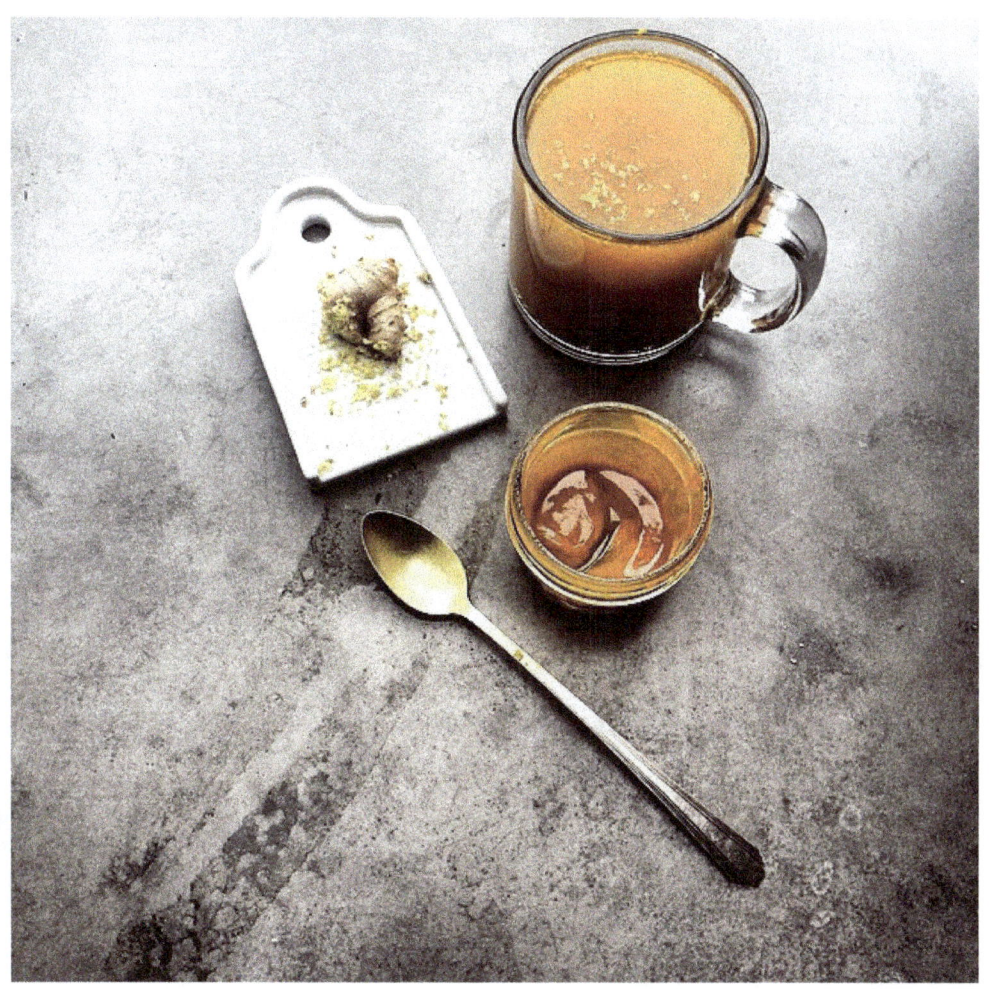

Turmeric Delight

Time To Prepare: five minutes
Time to Cook: 0 minutes
Yield: Servings 2

Ingredients:

- ¼ Teaspoon Ginger
- ½ Teaspoon Cinnamon
- 1 Banana, Sliced
- 1 Tablespoon Lemon Juice, Fresh
- 1 Teaspoon Turmeric
- 2 Cups Yogurt, Plain & Whole Milk
- 2 Teaspoons Honey, Raw

Directions:

Combine all ingredients into a blender then blend until the desired smoothness is achieved.

Nutritional Info: Calories: 234 ‖ Protein: 9.3 Grams ‖ Fat: 8.2 Grams ‖ Carbohydrates: 33.5 Grams

Turmeric Hot Chocolate

Time To Prepare: five minutes
Time to Cook: ten minutes
Yield: Servings 2

Ingredients:

- 1/8 tsp. cayenne pepper, optional
- 1/8 tsp. pepper
- 2 cups milk
- 2 tsp. ground turmeric
- 3 tbsp. cacao or cocoa powder
- 4 tsp. coconut oil
- 4 tsp. honey

Directions:

1. Put in milk, turmeric, cocoa, and coconut oil into a deep cooking pan. Put the deep cooking pan on moderate heat. Coconut oil and pepper are added because it helps to absorb the turmeric.
2. Whisk regularly until well blended.
3. When it starts to boil, remove from heat. Put in honey, cayenne pepper, and pepper and whisk well.
4. Split into 2 cups before you serve.

Nutritional Info: Calories: 339 kcal ‖ Protein: 12.76 g ‖ Fat: 21.19 g ‖ Carbohydrates: 30.35 g

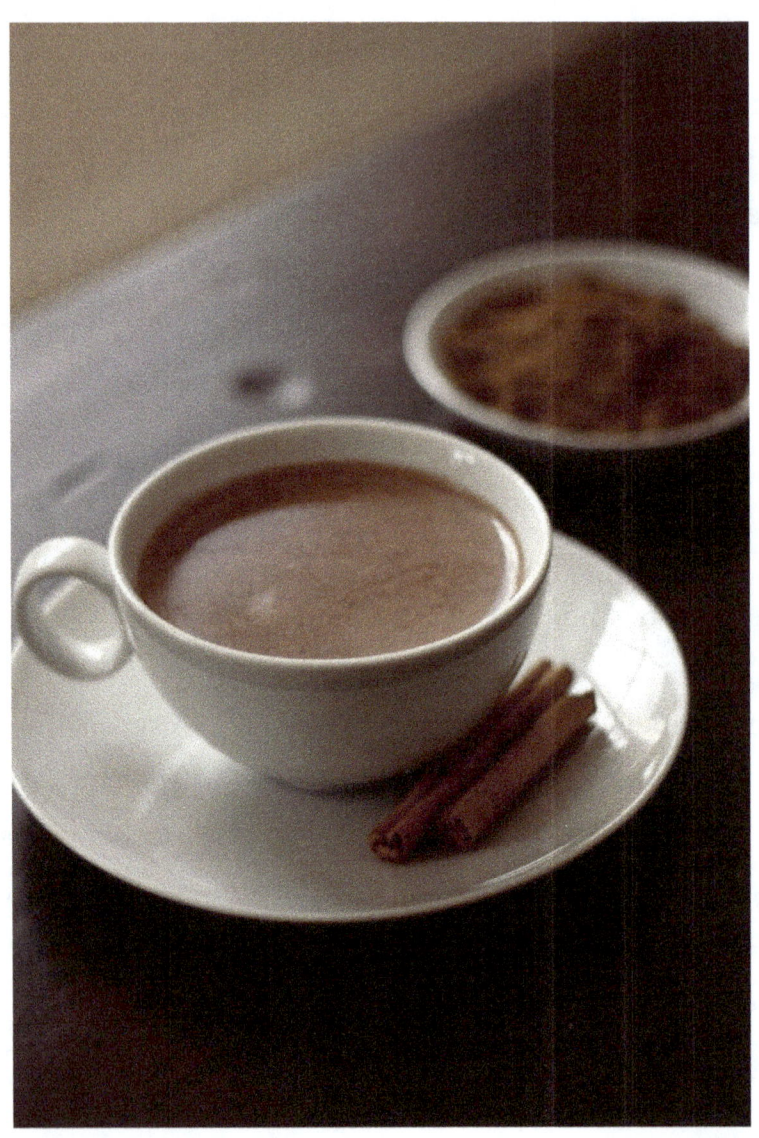

Turmeric Tea

Time To Prepare: five minutes
Time to Cook: fifteen minutes
Yield: Servings 2

Ingredients:

- ½ teaspoon ground ginger
- ½ teaspoon turmeric powder
- ½ tsp ground cinnamon
- 2 cups water
- 2 lemon juices
- 2 tablespoons honey

Directions:

1. Put in water into a deep cooking pan. Put the deep cooking pan on moderate heat.
2. When it starts to boil, put in turmeric, cinnamon, and ginger and stir slowly.
3. Remove the heat. Cover and allow the mixture to steep for 12 – fifteen minutes. Put in honey and lemon juice.
4. Stir and pour into mugs.
5. Serve.

Nutritional Info: Calories: 121 kcal ‖ Protein: 3.57 g ‖ Fat: 3.2 g ‖ Carbohydrates: 21.97 g

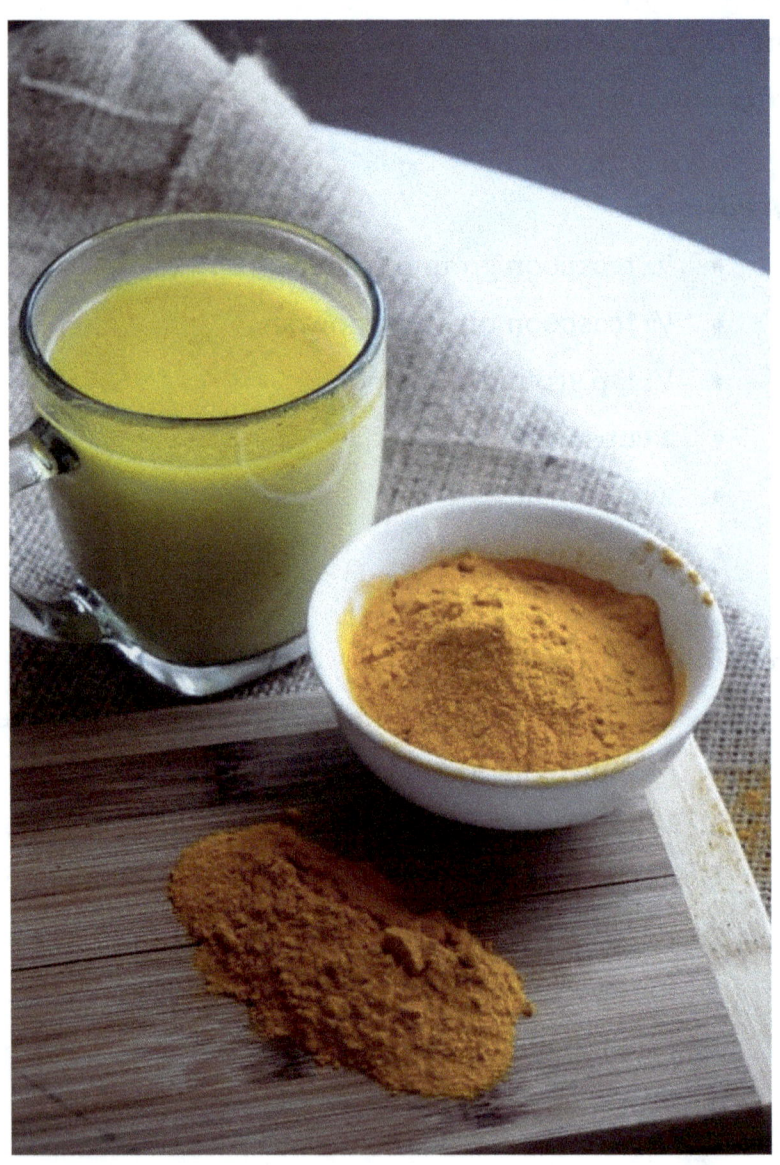

Vanilla Avocado Smoothie

Time To Prepare: ten minutes
Time to Cook: 0 minutes
Yield: Servings 1

Ingredients:
- 1 cup almond milk
- 1 ripe avocado, halved and pitted
- 1/2 cup vanilla yogurt
- 3 tbsp. honey
- 8 ice cubes

Directions:
1. Put in everything to a blender jug.
2. Cover the jug firmly.
3. Blend until the desired smoothness is achieved. Serve and enjoy!

Nutritional Info: Calories: 143 ‖ Fat: 1.2 g ‖ Protein: 4.6 g ‖ Carbohydrates: 21 g ‖ Fiber: 2.3 g

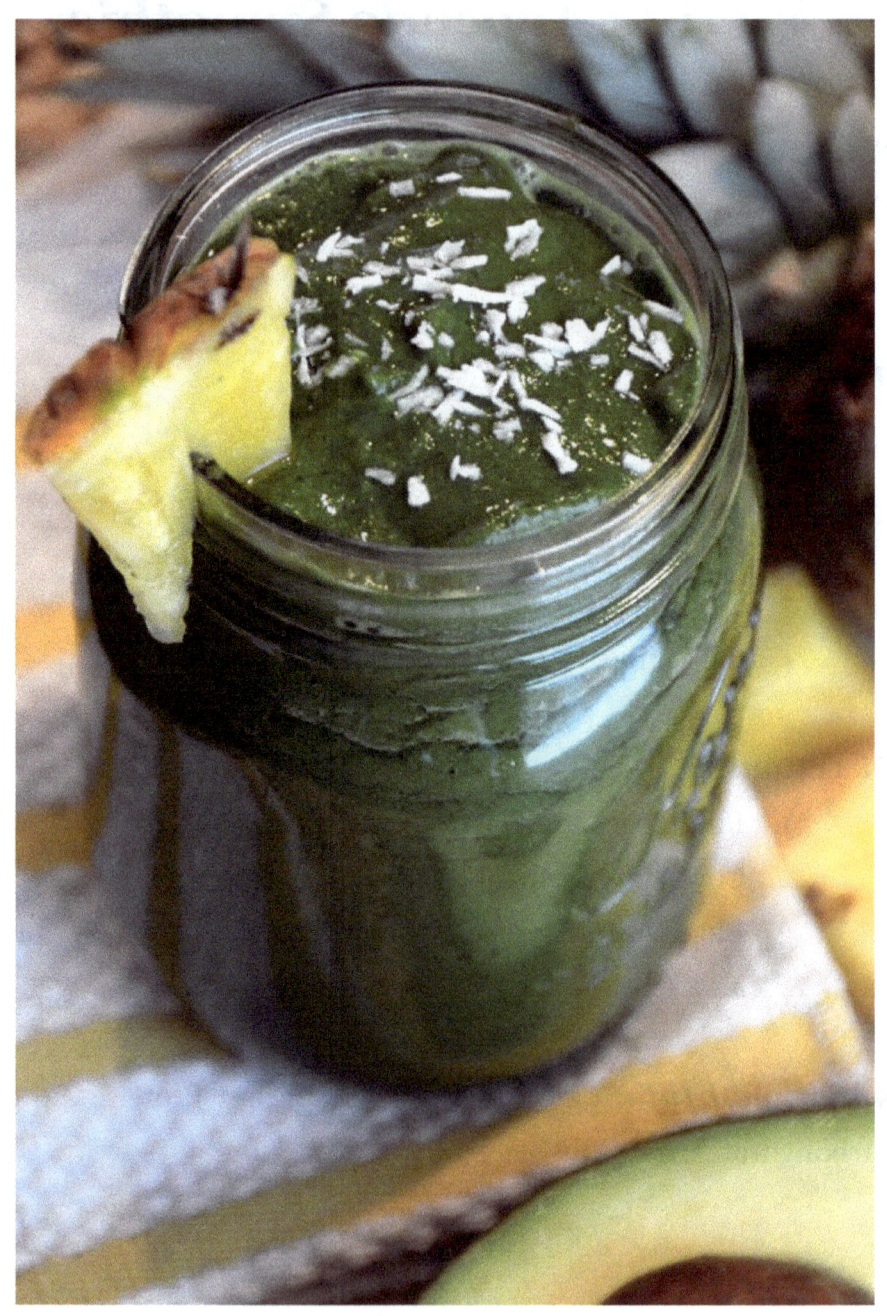

SIDES

Spicy Roasted Brussels Sprouts

Time To Prepare: five minutes
Time to Cook: thirty minutes
Yield: Servings 4

Ingredients:

- ½ cup kimchi with juice
- 1 and ¼ pound Brussels sprouts, cut into florets
- 2 tablespoons olive oil
- Salt and pepper, to taste

Directions:

1. Set the oven to 425 F.
2. Toss the Brussels sprouts with pepper, salt, and oil.
3. Bake using your oven for about twenty-five minutes
4. Remove from oven and mix with kimchi
5. Return to the oven
6. Cook for five minutes
7. Serve and enjoy!

Nutritional Info: ‖ Calories: 135 ‖ Fat: 7g ‖ Carbohydrates: 16g ‖ Protein: 5g

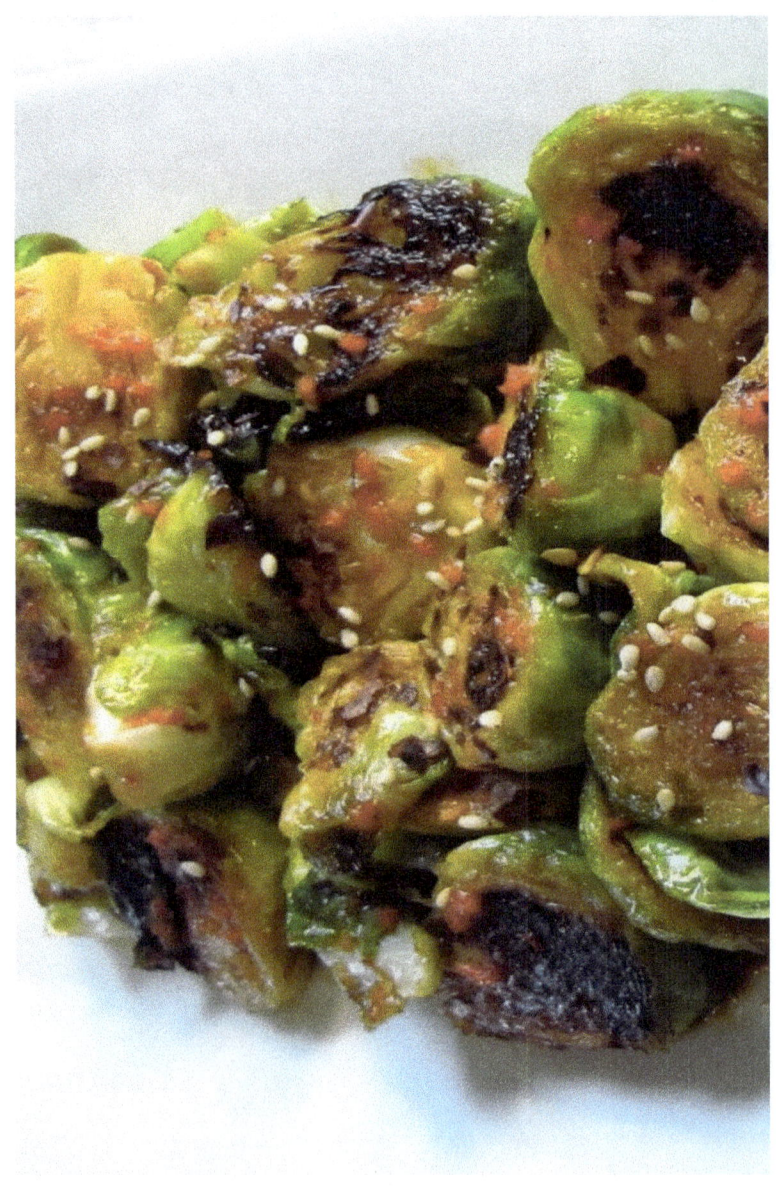

Spicy Wasabi Mayonnaise

Time To Prepare: fifteen minutes
Time to Cook: 0 minute
Yield: Servings 4

Ingredients:
- ½ tablespoon wasabi paste
- 1 cup mayonnaise

Directions:
1. Take a container and mix wasabi paste and mayonnaise

Mix thoroughly

2. Allow it to chill, use as required
3. Serve and enjoy

Nutritional Info: ‖ Calories: 388 ‖ Fat: 42g ‖ Carbohydrates: 1g ‖ Protein: 1g

Stir-Fried Almond And Spinach

Time To Prepare: ten minutes
Time to Cook: fifteen minutes
Yield: Servings 2

Ingredients:
- 1 tablespoon coconut oil
- 3 tablespoons almonds
- 34 pounds spinach
- Salt to taste

Directions:
1. Put oil to a big pot and place it on high heat
2. Put in spinach and allow it to cook, stirring regularly
3. Once the spinach is cooked and soft, sprinkle with salt and stir
4. Put in almonds and enjoy!

Nutritional Info: ‖ Calories: 150 ‖ Fat: 12g ‖ Carbohydrates: 10g ‖ Protein: 8g

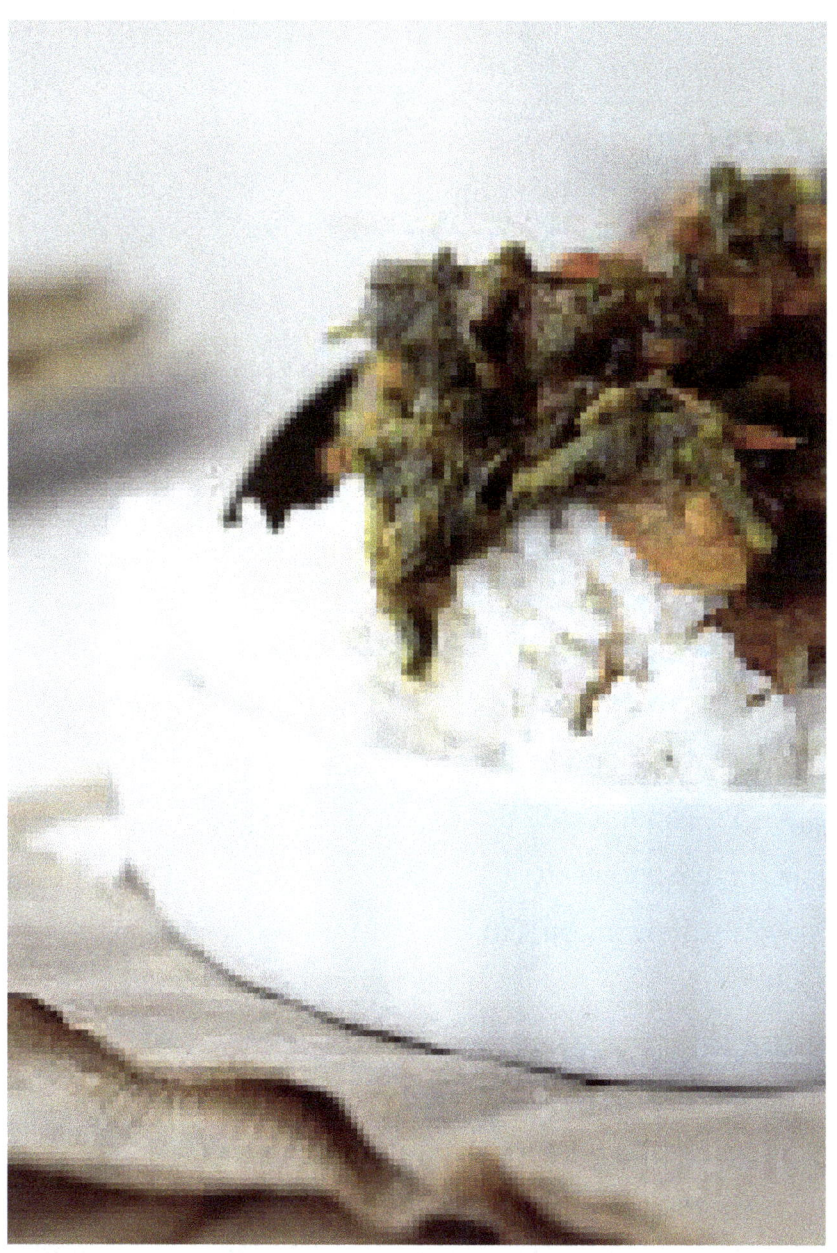

Stir-Fried Farros

Time To Prepare: five minutes
Time to Cook: thirty-five minutes
Yield: Servings 2

Ingredients:

- ½ cup farro
- ½ teaspoon ground coriander
- ½ teaspoon paprika
- ½ teaspoon turmeric
- 1 ½ cup water
- 1 carrot, grated
- 1 tablespoon butter
- 1 teaspoon chili flakes
- 1 teaspoon salt
- 1 yellow onion, cut

Directions:

1. Put farro in the pan. Put in water and salt.
2. Close the lid and boil it for half an hour
3. In the meantime, toss the butter in the frying pan.
4. Heat it and put in cut onion and grated carrot.

5. Fry the vegetables for about ten minutes over the moderate heat. Stir them with the help of spatula occasionally.
6. When the farro is cooked, put in it in the roasted vegetables and mix up well.
7. Cook stir-fried farro for five minutes over the moderate to high heat.

Nutritional Info: Calories 129 ‖ Fat: 5.9 ‖ Fiber: 3 ‖ Carbs: 17.1 ‖ Protein: 2.8

SAUCES AND DRESSINGS

Strawberry Poppy Seed Dressing

Time To Prepare: ten minutes
Time to Cook: 0 minutes
Yield: Servings 2-4

Ingredients:

- ¼ cup of raspberry vinegar
- ¼ tsp of ground ginger
- ¼ tsp of sea salt
- ½ tsp of onion powder
- ½ tsp of poppy seeds
- 1/3 cup of extra-virgin olive oil
- 1/3 cup of honey
- 2 tbsp. of freshly squeezed orange juice

Directions:

1. Put all ingredients, apart from the poppy seeds and oil into a blender. Blend until the desired smoothness is achieved and creamy. Next, progressively put the oil

into the mixture until blended. Put in in the poppy seeds and stir thoroughly.
2. Put in a mason jar then place in your fridge before you serve. Keep for maximum 3 days.
3. Serve with your garden salads.

Nutritional Info: ‖ Calories: 167 kcal ‖ Protein: 1.84 g ‖ Fat: 9.35 g ‖ Carbohydrates: 18.89 g

Tahini Dip

Time To Prepare: ten minutes
Time to Cook: 0 minutes
Yield: Servings 2-4

Ingredients:

- ¼ cup of tahini
- ½ tsp of maple syrup
- 1 small grated or thoroughly minced clove of garlic (this is optional)
- 1 tbsp. of apple cider vinegar
- 1 tbsp. of freshly squeezed lemon juice
- 1 tbsp. of tamari
- 1 tsp of finely grated ginger, or ½ tsp of ground ginger
- 1 tsp of turmeric
- 1/3 cup of water

Directions:

1. Blend or whisk all ingredients together. Place the dressing in an airtight container then place in your fridge for approximately 5 days.
2. Enjoy!

Nutritional Info: ‖ Calories: 120 kcal ‖ Protein: 4.77 g ‖ Fat: 9.63 g ‖ Carbohydrates: 5.12 g

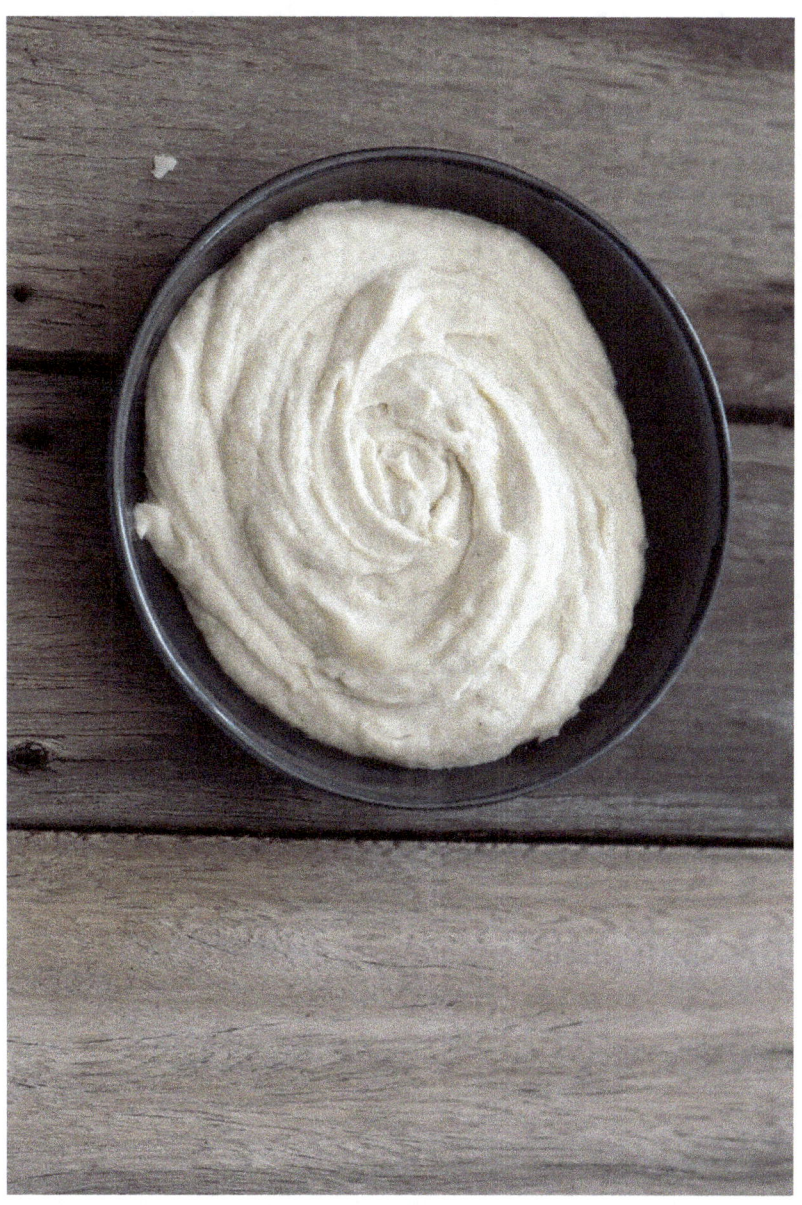

SNACKS

Roasted Garlic Chickpeas

Time To Prepare: five minutes
Time to Cook: twenty minutes
Yield: Servings 2

Ingredients:

- 1 Teaspoon Garlic Powder
- 1 Teaspoon Sea Salt
- 2 Tablespoons Olive Oil
- 4 Cups Cooked Chickpeas, Rinsed, Drained & Dried
- Black Pepper to Taste

Directions:

1. Begin by heating the oven to 400.
2. Spread your chickpeas on a baking sheet, coating them with your olive oil.
3. Bake of 20 minutes, ensuring to stir them at the ten-minute mark.
4. Put your hot chickpeas in a container, seasoning before securing them in an airtight container. They'll keep at room temperature for maximum two days.

Nutritional Info: ‖ Calories: 150 ‖ Protein: 6 Grams ‖ Fat: 5 Grams ‖ Carbohydrates: 21 Grams

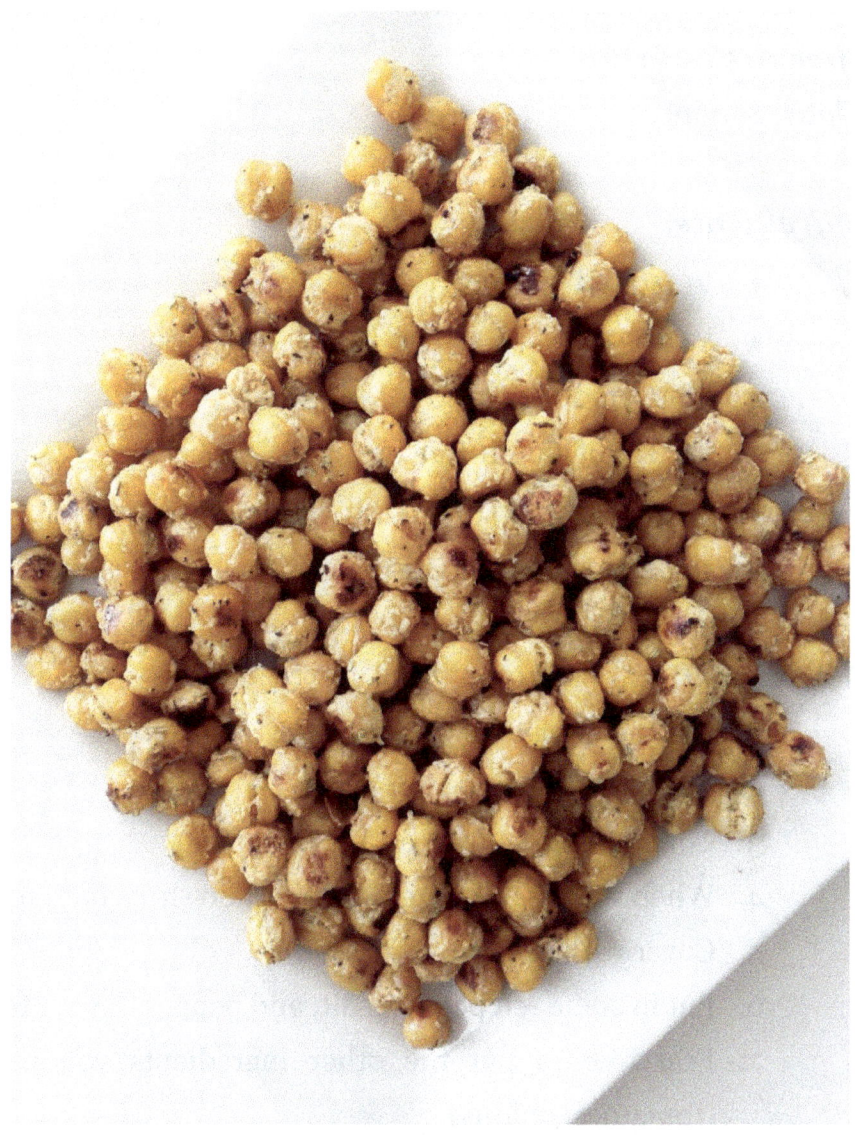

Salmon & Avocado Toast

Time To Prepare: ten minutes
Time to Cook: five minutes
Yield: Servings 1

Ingredients:

- ¼ tsp red pepper
- ½ avocado
- 1 tsp lemon juice
- 2 slices of gluten-free bread
- oz. pink salmon (wild)
- salt and pepper - to taste

Directions:

1. Cut the avocado.
2. Toast the bread to your taste.
3. Combine the salmon and lemon juice.
4. When the toast is ready, lay avocado slices onto it.
5. Cover with salmon.
6. Put in some red pepper, salt, and pepper to your taste.
7. Feel free to put the other ingredients you prefer (tomatoes, onions)
8. Enjoy your salmon snack!

Nutritional Info: ‖ Calories: 481 kcal ‖ Protein: 28.08 g ‖ Fat: 27.52 g ‖ Carbohydrates: 33 g

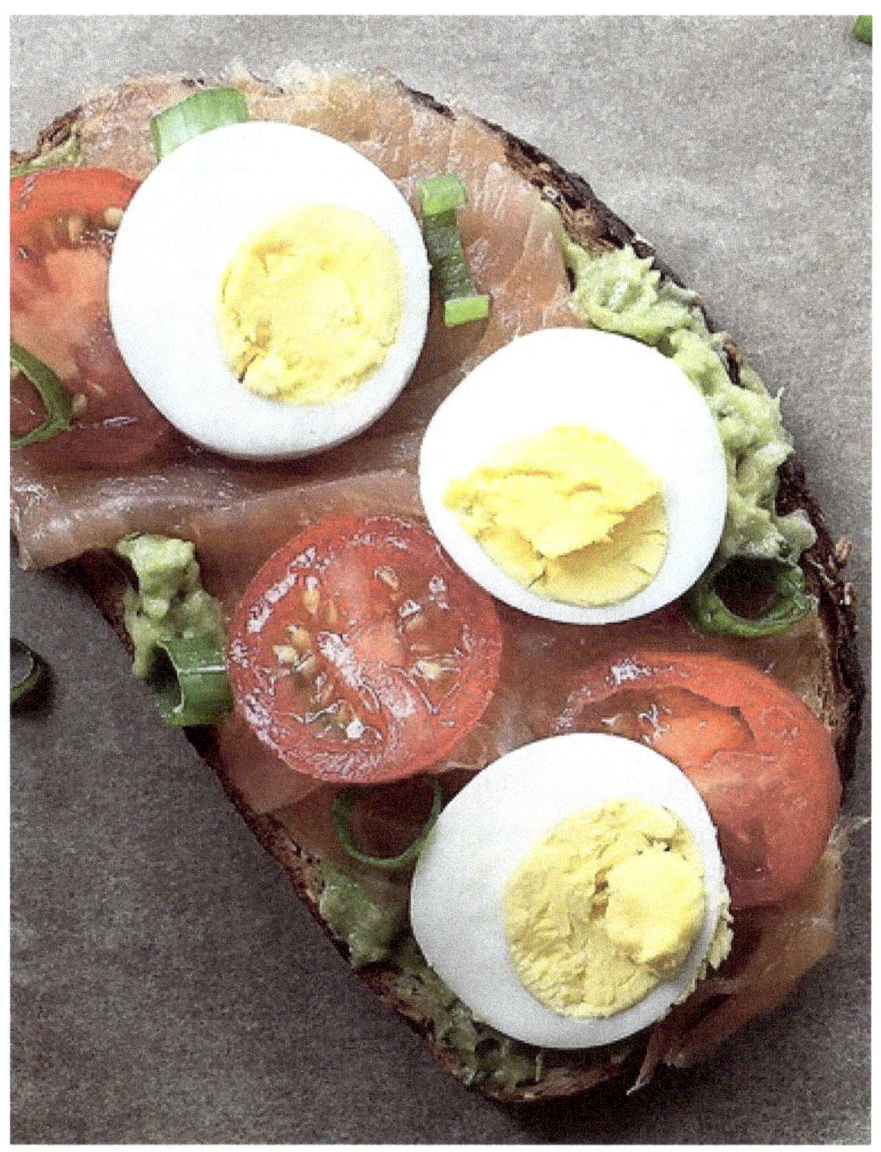

Salt & Vinegar Kale Crisps

Time To Prepare: five minutes
Time to Cook: 20-twenty-five minutes
Yield: Servings 2

Ingredients:

- 1 Teaspoon Sea Salt, Fine
- 2 Tablespoon Apple Cider Vinegar
- 2 Tablespoons Olive Oil
- 4 Cups Kale, Torn into 2 Inch Pieces

Directions:

1. Begin by heating the oven to 350. Get out a container, and mix all of your ingredients.
2. Put your kale on a baking sheet, baking for twenty to twenty-five minutes. Toss midway through this time.
3. Put at room temperature in an airtight container. They'll keep for two days.

Nutritional Info: ‖ Calories: 135 ‖ Protein: 1 Gram ‖ Fat: 14 Grams ‖ Carbohydrates: 3 Grams

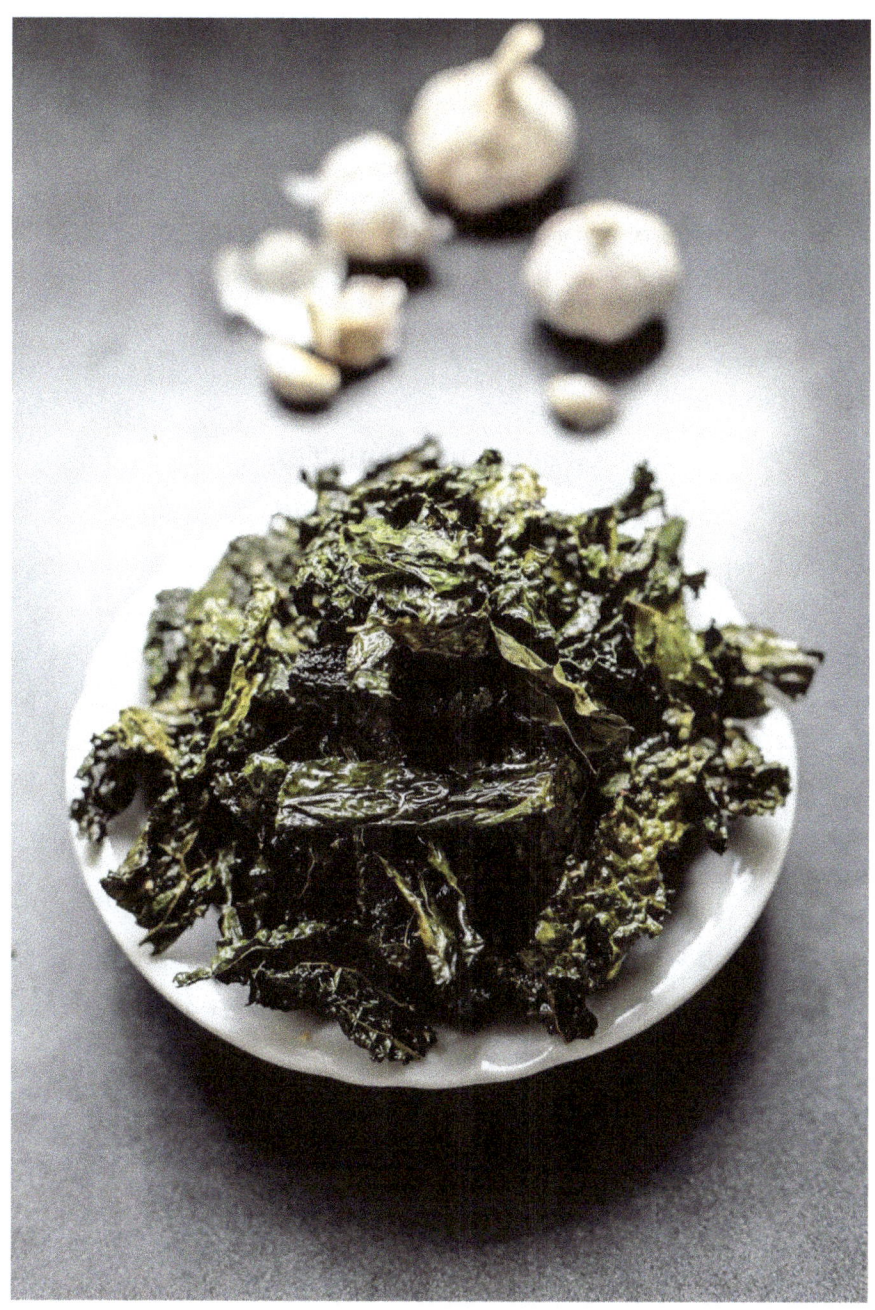

Soft Flourless Cookies

Time To Prepare: ten minutes
Time to Cook: twenty-five minutes
Yield: Servings 4

Ingredients:

- ¼ teaspoon of organic vanilla extract
- ¾ cup of shredded unsweetened coconut
- 1 peeled big banana
- Pinch of ground cinnamon

Directions:

1. Set the oven to 350F. Coat a cookie sheet with a big greased parchment paper.
2. In a big food processor, put all ingredients and pulse till well blended.
3. Ladle the mixture onto the prepared cookie sheet. Use your hands to flatten the cookies slightly.
4. Bake for minimum twenty-five minutes or till golden brown.

Nutritional Info: ‖ Calories: 84 ‖ Fat: 5.1g ‖ Carbohydrates: 10.1g ‖ Protein: 0.9g ‖ Fiber: 2.3g

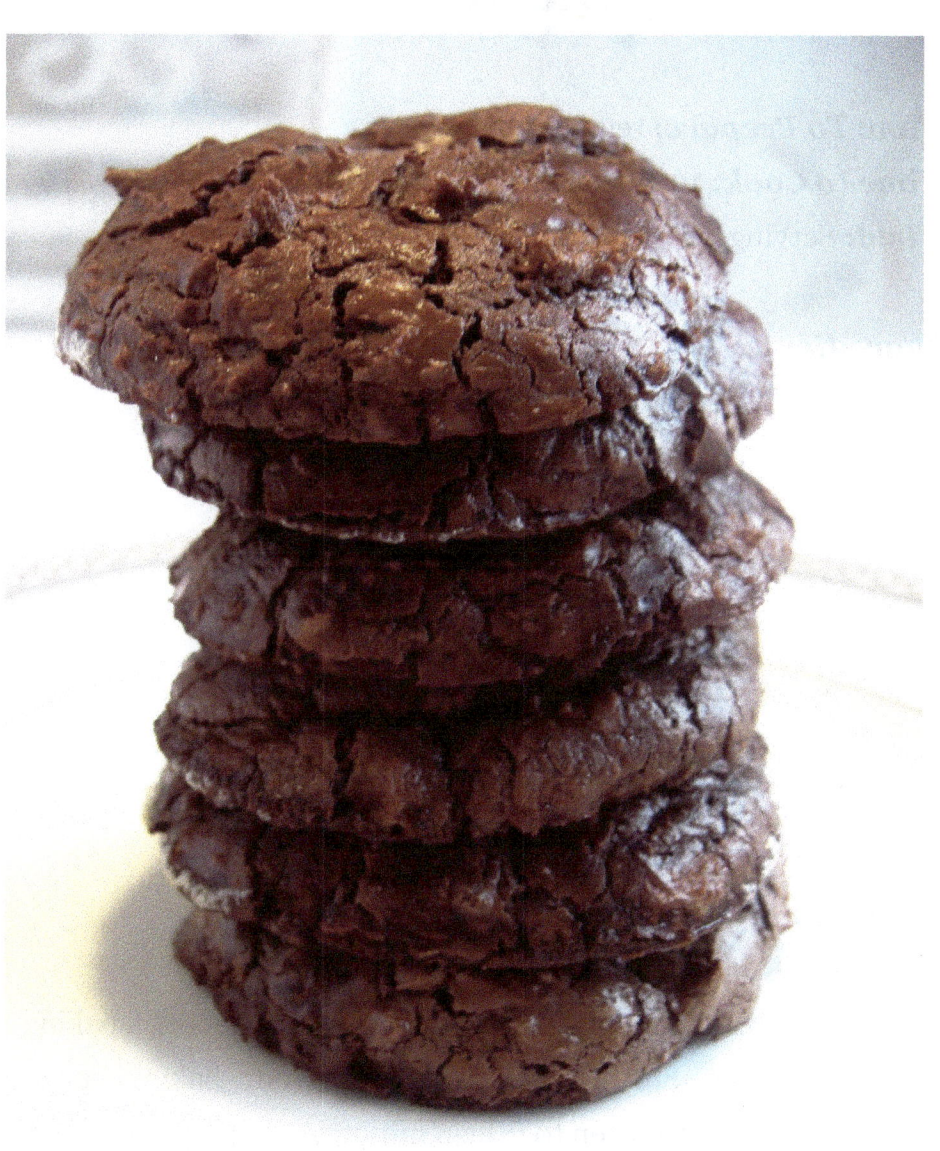

Spiced Nuts

Time To Prepare: ten minutes
Time to Cook: 10-fifteen minutes
Yield: Servings 2

Ingredients:

- ¼ Cup Pumpkin Puree
- ¼ Cup Sunflower Seeds
- ¼ Teaspoon Garlic Powder
- ¼ Teaspoon Red Pepper Flakes
- ½ Cup Walnuts
- ½ Teaspoon Ground Cumin
- 1 Cup Almonds
- 1 Teaspoon Ground Turmeric

Directions:

1. Begin by heating the oven to 350.
2. Mix all ingredients together, and then get out a baking sheet. Spread your nuts over your baking sheet, cooking for ten to fifteen minutes.
3. Allow it to cool well before you store it.

Nutritional Info: ‖ Calories: 180 ‖ Protein: 6 Grams ‖ Fat: 16 Grams ‖ Carbohydrates: 7 Grams

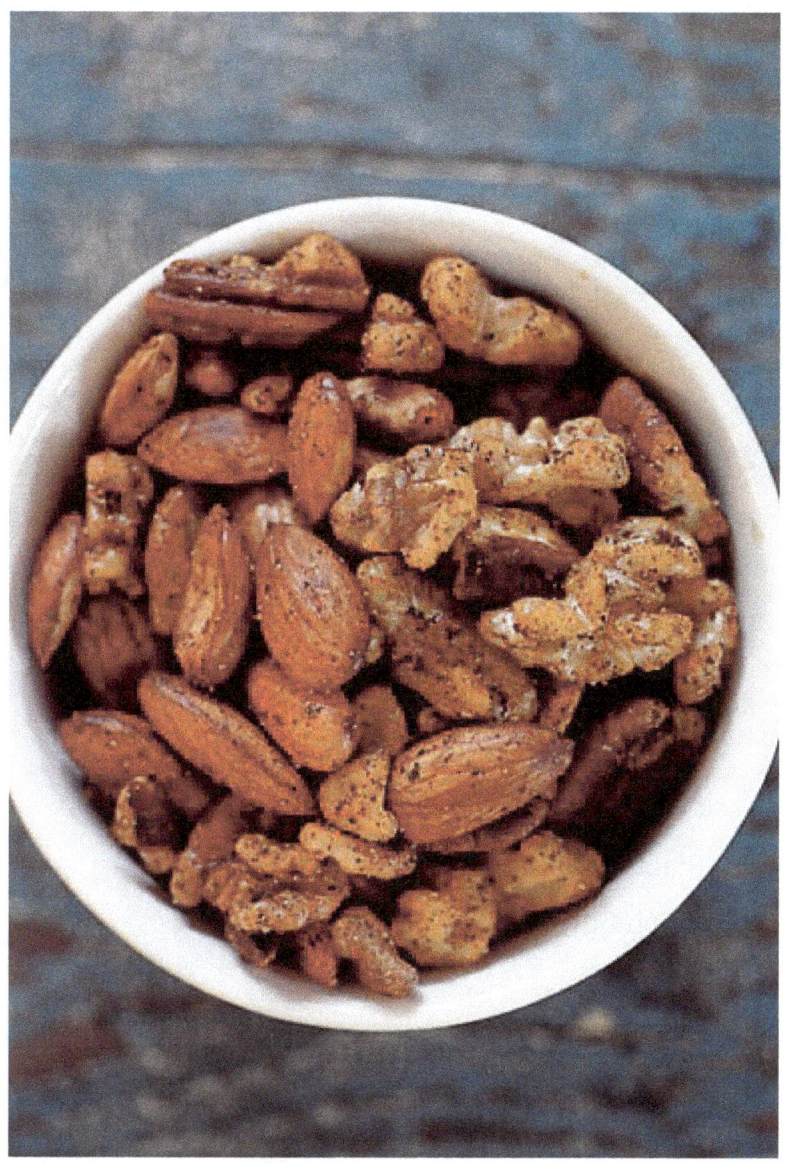

Spicy Bean Dip

Time To Prepare: ten minutes
Time to Cook: 0 minutes
Yield: Servings 3

Ingredients:

- ¼ Teaspoon Ground Cumin
- ¼ Teaspoon Sea Salt
- 1 Tablespoon Apple Cider Vinegar
- 1 Teaspoon Lime Juice, Fresh
- 14 Ounce Can Black Beans, Drained & Rinsed
- 14 Ounce Can Kidney Beans, Drained & Rinsed
- 2 Cherry Tomatoes
- 2 Cloves Garlic
- 2 Tablespoons Water
- 2 Teaspoon Honey, Raw
- Black Pepper to Taste
- Pinch Cayenne Pepper

Directions:

1. Mix all of your ingredients in a food processor, and blend until it's smooth.
2. Cover, and place in your fridge before you serve.

Nutritional Info: ‖ Calories: 166 ‖ Protein: 9.4 Grams ‖ Fat: 0.6 Grams ‖ Carbohydrates: 34.2 Grams

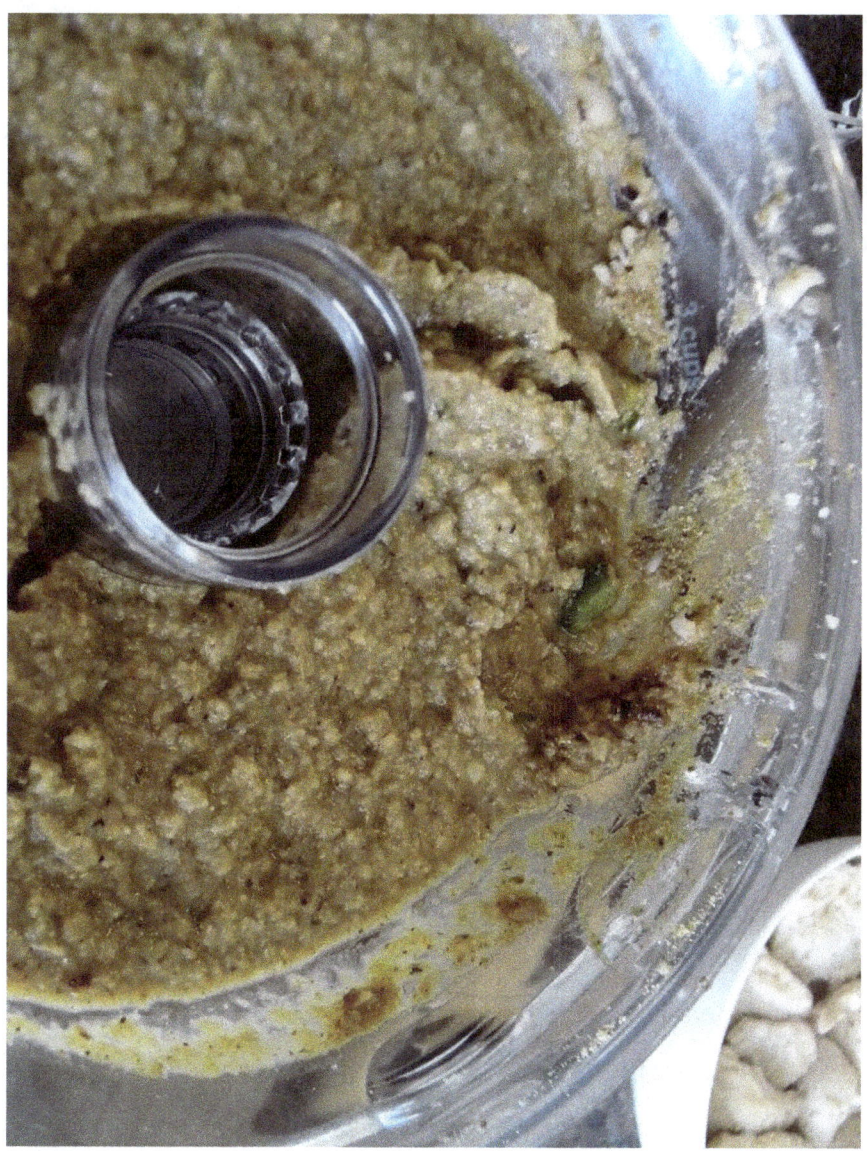

Spicy Roasted chickpeas

Time To Prepare: ten minutes
Time to Cook: forty minutes
Yield: Servings 6

Ingredients:

- ¼ teaspoon of cayenne pepper
- 1 teaspoon of paprika
- 1 teaspoon of turmeric
- 2 (fifteen ounce) cans of chickpeas, drained and washed
- 2 teaspoons of coconut oil, melted

Directions:

1. Set the oven to 425°F.
2. Coat a baking sheet using a paper towels, then put the chickpeas on them and use more paper towels to take off the surplus water in the chickpeas. Remove all of the paper towels.
3. Place the oil and spices to the chickpeas and mix thoroughly.
4. Roast your chickpeas for forty minutes, stirring every ten minutes.

5. Once the chickpeas are done, take it off from the oven and let fully cool.

Nutritional Info: ‖ Total Carbohydrates: 19g ‖ Fiber: 6g ‖ Net Carbohydrates: ‖ Protein: 7g ‖ Total Fat: 4g ‖ Calories: 138

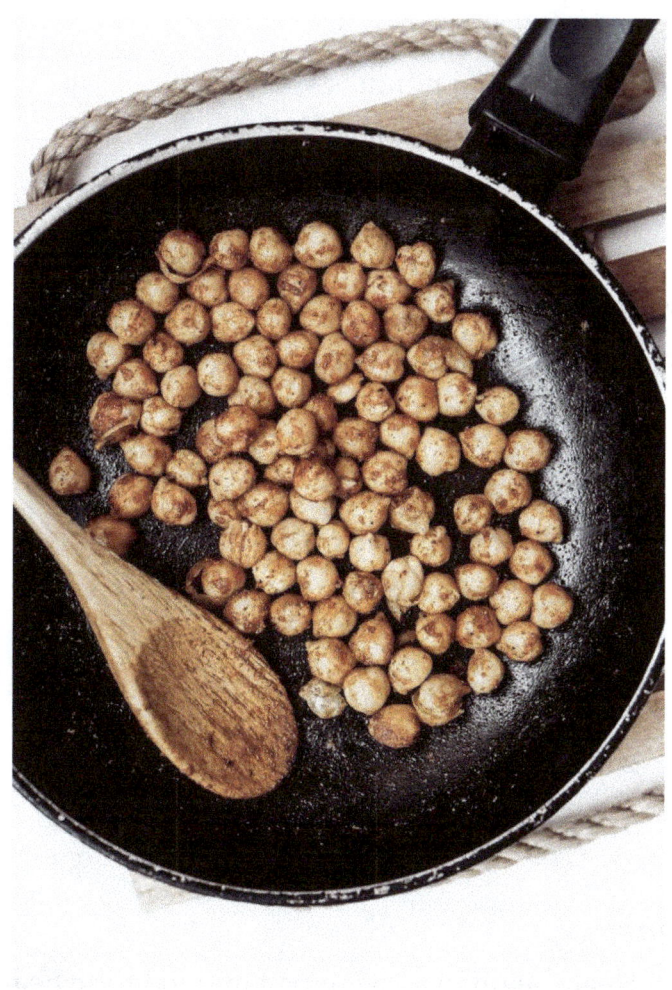

SOUPS AND STEWS

Spicy Cabbage Turmeric Coconut Soup

Time To Prepare: ten minutes
Time to Cook: twenty minutes
Yield: Servings 4

Ingredients:

- ½ teaspoon black pepper
- ½ teaspoon salt
- 1 head white cabbage
- 1 teaspoon cumin powder
- 1/4 cup coconut milk
- 2 cloves garlic
- 2 tablespoons coconut oil
- 2 teaspoons turmeric powder
- 3 cups vegetable/chicken stock

Directions:

1. Heat the oil in a frying pan on moderate heat.

2. Put in the cabbage & garlic & sauté until the cabbage is delicate.
3. Put in the stock, bubble, spread, & stew for about twenty minutes.
4. Turn off the heat, including the coconut milk & flavors.
5. Blend until the desired smoothness is achieved & season to taste. Serve, gulp & appreciate!

Nutritional Info: Calories: 207 kcal ‖ Protein: 13.52 g ‖ Fat: 10.79 g ‖ Carbohydrates: 16.84 g

Spicy Lime-Chicken "Tortilla-Less" Soup

Time To Prepare: ten minutes
Time to Cook: twenty minutes
Yield: Servings 6

Ingredients:

- ¼ teaspoon cayenne pepper
- ½ teaspoon salt
- 1 (14 oz.) can diced tomatoes, and it's juice
- 1 (4oz.) can diced green chiles
- 1 avocado, cut
- 1 jalapeño pepper, seeded and minced
- 1 medium white onion, diced
- 1 pound shredded cooked chicken
- 1 tablespoon avocado oil
- 1 teaspoon chili powder
- 1 teaspoon ground cumin
- 3 garlic cloves, minced
- 3 tablespoons freshly squeezed lime juice
- 6 cups chicken broth or vegetable broth
- Fresh cilantro, for decoration

- Freshly ground black pepper

Directions:

1. In a huge soup pot on moderate heat, heat the avocado oil.
2. Put in the garlic, onion, and jalapeño pepper, and sauté for five minutes.
3. Mix in the broth, chicken, tomatoes, green chiles, lime juice, chili powder, cumin, salt, and cayenne pepper, and flavor with black pepper. Put it to a simmer, and cook for about ten minutes.
4. Serve hot, topped with slices of avocado and decorated with cilantro.

Nutritional Info: Calories: 283 ‖ Total Fat: 7g ‖ Saturated Fat: 1g ‖ Cholesterol: 47mg ‖ Carbohydrates: 12g ‖ Fiber: 3g ‖ Protein: 29g

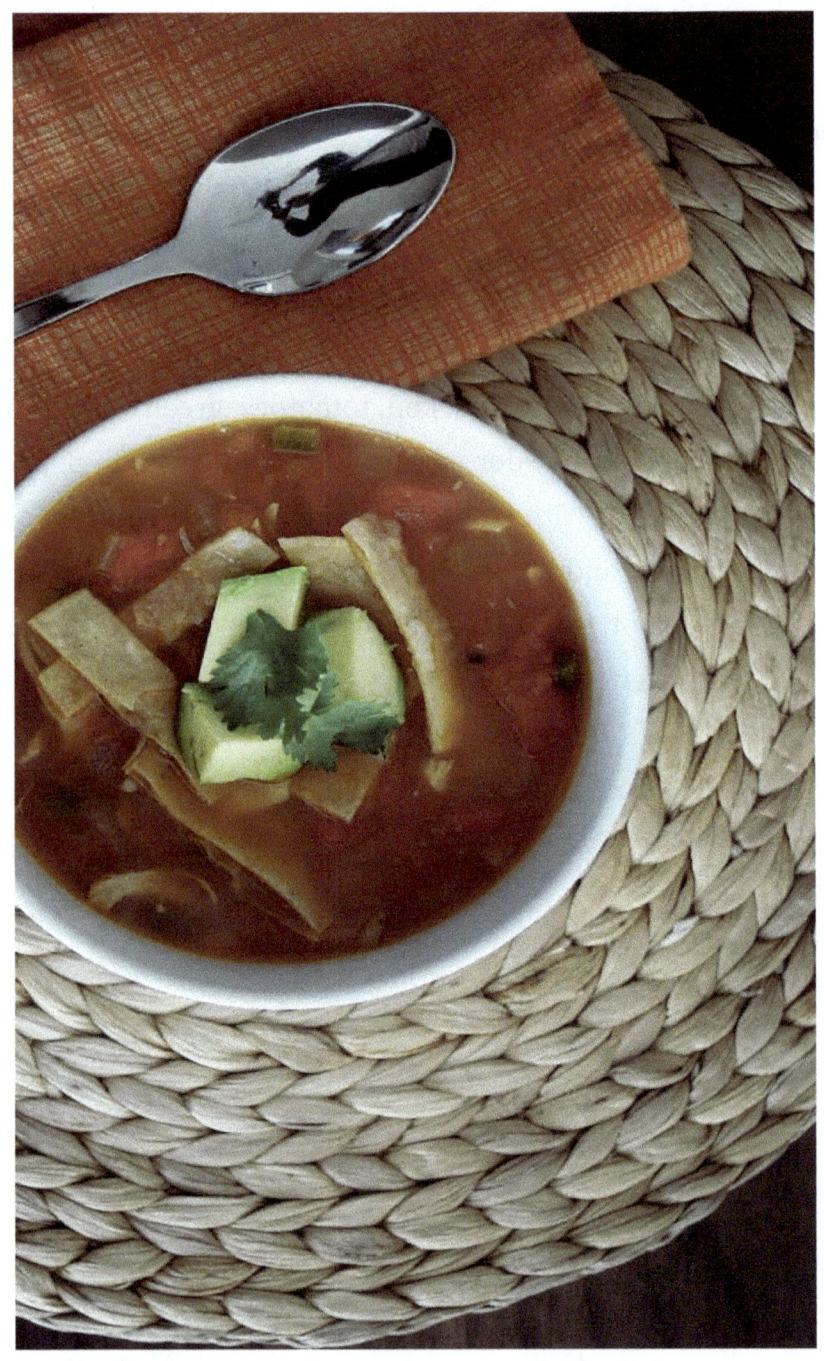

Spicy Ramen Noodles

Time To Prepare: fifteen minutes
Time to Cook: 0 minutes
Yield: Servings 4

Ingredients:

- ¼ cup chopped fresh cilantro
- ¼ cup cut scallion
- ¼ cup thinly cut cucumber
- 1 tablespoon coconut aminos
- 1 tablespoon freshly squeezed lime juice
- 1 tablespoon grated peeled fresh ginger
- 1 tablespoon raw honey
- 1 teaspoon chili powder
- 2 tablespoons rice vinegar
- 2 tablespoons sesame oil
- 2 tablespoons sesame seeds
- 8 ounces buckwheat noodles or rice noodles, cooked

Directions:

1. In a big serving container, meticulously mix the noodles, sesame seeds, cucumber, scallion, cilantro,

sesame oil, vinegar, ginger, coconut aminos, honey, lime juice, and chili powder.
2. Split among 4 soup bowls and serve at room temperature.

Nutritional Info: Calories: 663 ∥ Total Fat: 28g ∥ Saturated Fat: 4g ∥ Cholesterol: 0mg ∥ Carbohydrates: 115g ∥ Fiber: 39g ∥ Protein: 21g

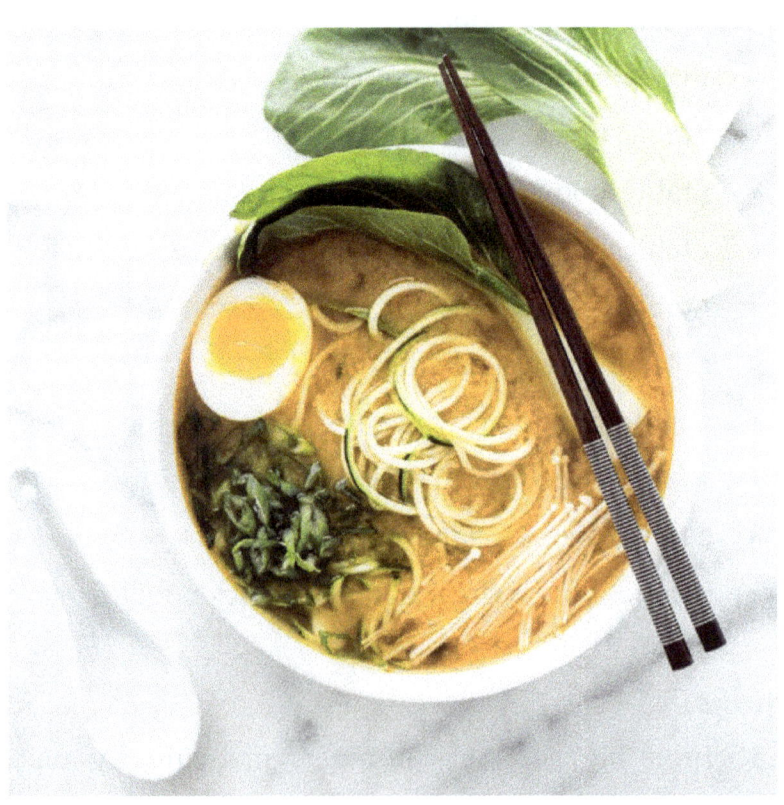

Spicy Seafood Stew

Time To Prepare: ten minutes
Time to Cook: twenty minutes
Yield: Servings 6

Ingredients:

- ¼ cup freshly squeezed lime juice
- ½ cup chopped fresh cilantro
- ½ cup chopped yellow onion
- ½ cup coconut milk
- ½ cup diced green pepper
- ½ cup thinly cut scallions
- ¾ pound medium-size shrimp, shelled and deveined
- ¾ pound skinless firm-fleshed fish fillets, (cod, center-cut salmon, or halibut)
- 1 tablespoon minced garlic
- 1 teaspoon hot pepper sauce
- 2 tablespoons olive oil
- 3 cups canned peeled, chopped tomatoes, undrained
- Seasoned salt, to taste

Directions:

1. Warm the oil in a huge nonstick frying pan on moderate to high heat. Put in the onions, green pepper, garlic, and tomatoes. Put to a simmer while stirring once in a while, then cook for three to four minutes.
2. Put in the coconut milk, pepper sauce, lime juice, and seasoned salt. Set to a simmer and cook for minimum 2 minutes. Put in the fish and stir, being cautious not to break apart the fillets. Cook till the fish is thoroughly cooked, approximately eight minutes. Put in the shrimp and cook until opaque and thoroughly cooked, approximately five minutes.
3. To serve, use a slotted spoon to take equal amounts of the fish and shrimp to 4 shallow serving bowls. Place the sauce over the seafood and decorate with scallions and cilantro. Serve hot.

Nutritional Info: Calories: 219 ‖ Fat: 11 g ‖ Protein: 19g ‖ Sodium: 375 mg ‖ Fiber: 2 g ‖ Carbohydrates: 10 g

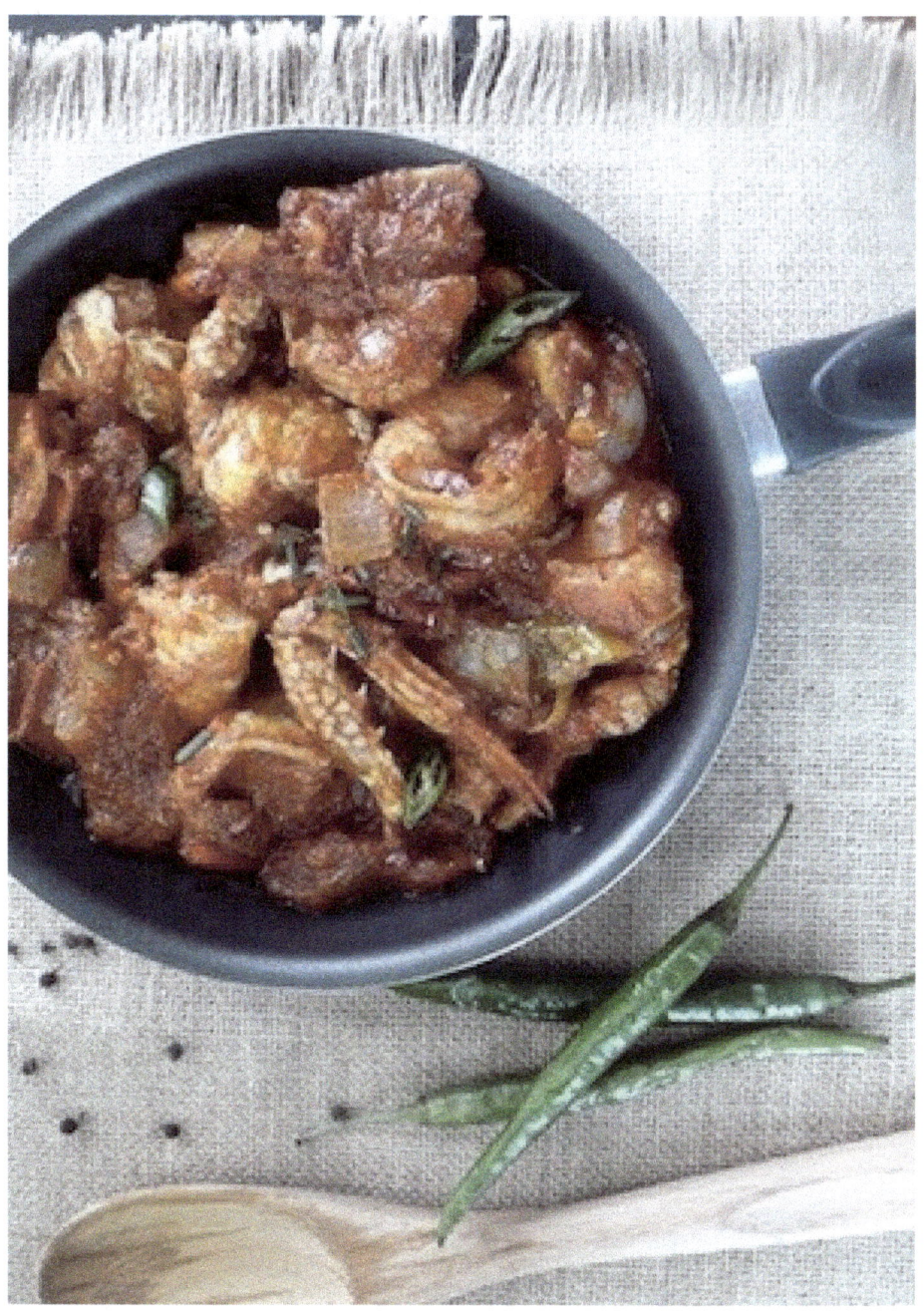

Sweet Potato and Black Bean Chili

Time To Prepare: ten minutes
Time to Cook: twenty minutes
Yield: Servings 8

Ingredients:

- ¼ teaspoon cayenne pepper
- ¼ teaspoon dried oregano
- ½ teaspoon ground cinnamon
- 1 (28-ounce) can diced tomatoes with their juice
- 1 green bell pepper, diced
- 1 red bell pepper, diced
- 1 red onion, diced
- 1 tablespoon chili powder
- 1 tablespoon freshly squeezed lime juice
- 1 teaspoon cocoa powder
- 1 teaspoon ground cumin
- 1 teaspoon salt
- 2 cups vegetable broth
- 2 tablespoons avocado oil
- 3 cups black beans, drained and washed well

- 3 cups cooked sweet potato cubes
- 5 garlic cloves, minced

Directions:

1. In a huge soup pot on moderate heat, warm the avocado oil.
2. Place the onion and garlic, and sauté for a couple of minutes.
3. Mix in the red bell pepper and the green bell pepper, and sauté for approximately 3 minutes until tender.
4. Put in the sweet potato, beans, broth, tomatoes, lime juice, chili powder, cocoa powder, cumin, salt, cinnamon, cayenne pepper, and oregano, then stir until blended. Put to a simmer, and cook for fifteen minutes. Serve instantly.

Nutritional Info: Calories: 160 ‖ Total Fat: 4g ‖ Saturated Fat: 0g ‖ Cholesterol: 0mg ‖ Carbohydrates: 29g ‖ Fiber: 6g ‖ Protein: 8g

Sweet Potato and Corn Soup

Time To Prepare: ten minutes
Time to Cook: twenty minutes
Yield: Servings 4

Ingredients:

- ¼ cup extra-virgin olive oil or coconut oil
- ¼ teaspoon freshly ground black pepper
- 1 cup broccoli florets
- 1 cup coconut milk or almond milk
- 1 cup frozen corn kernels
- 1 cup thinly cut mushrooms
- 1 medium zucchini, cut into ¼-inch dice
- 1 small onion, cut into ¼-inch dice
- 1 teaspoon salt
- 2 cups peeled sweet potatoes cut into ¼-inch dice
- 2 tablespoons finely chopped fresh flat-leaf parsley
- 4 cups vegetable broth

Directions:

1. In a large pot, heat the oil on high heat.
2. Put in the zucchini, broccoli, mushrooms, and onion and sauté until tender, 5 to 8 minutes.

3. Pour the broth and sweet potatoes and place it to its boiling point.
4. Lower the heat to a simmer and cook until the sweet potatoes are soft, five to seven minutes.
5. Put in the corn, coconut milk, parsley, salt, and pepper. Cook on low heat up to the corn is thoroughly heated before you serve.

Nutritional Info: Calories: 402 ‖ Total Fat: 29g ‖ Total Carbohydrates: 31g ‖ Sugar: 9g ‖ Fiber: 6g ‖ Protein: 10g ‖ Sodium: 1406mg

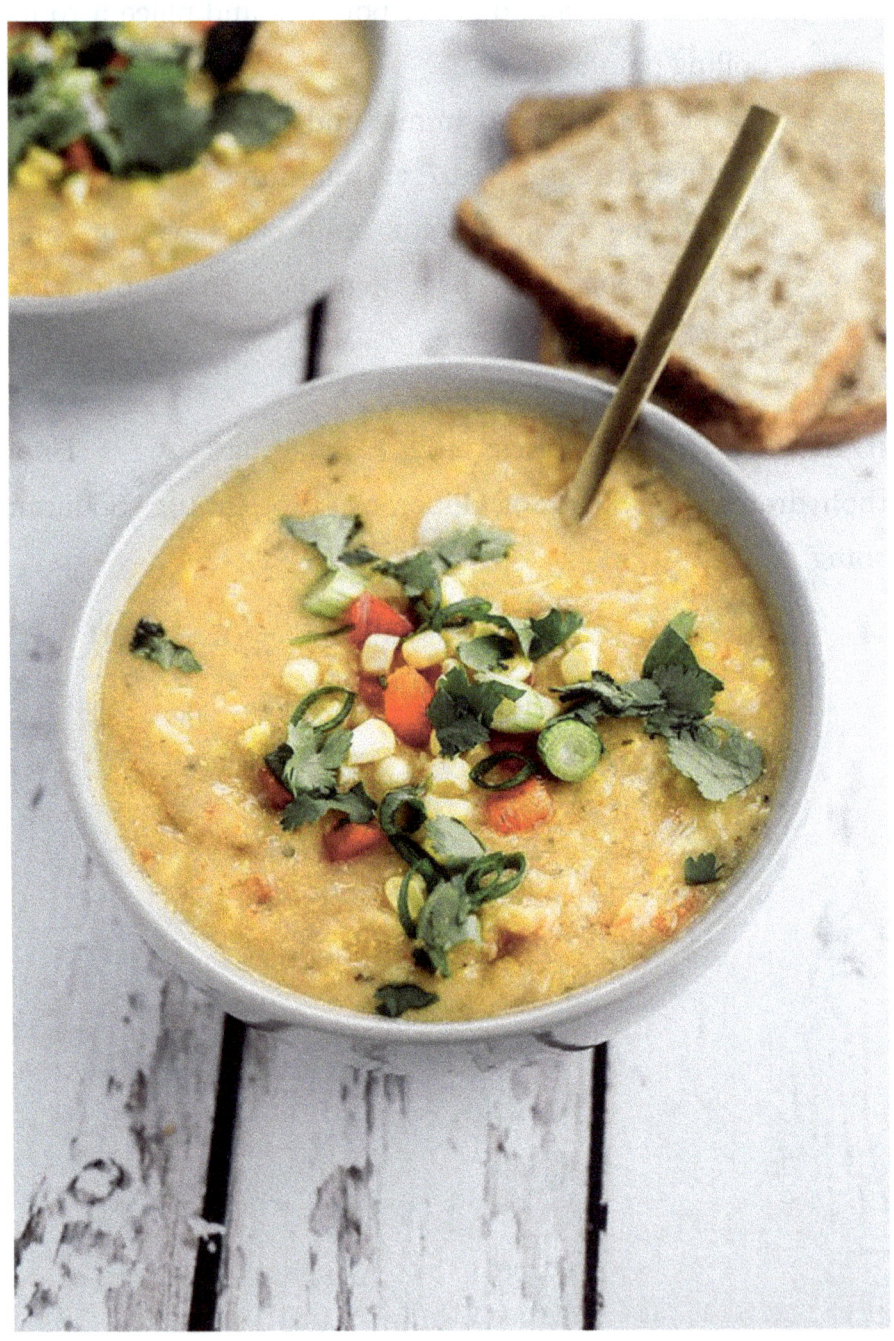

Tex-Mex Chicken Soup

Time To Prepare: ten minutes
Time to Cook: 1 hour
Yield: Servings 4

Ingredients:

- ¼ cup roasted pumpkin seeds
- 1 teaspoon paprika powder
- 1 yellow onion, chopped
- 1¾ cups coconut cream
- 12 ounces (340 g) boneless chicken thighs
- 2 tablespoons coconut oil
- 3 tablespoons Tex-Mex seasoning
- 4 tablespoons lime juice
- Fresh cilantro, chopped
- Salt and ground black pepper, to taste

Directions:

1. Cook the chicken thighs in a pot of water, covered, for thirty minutes or until the chicken is completely fork-soft. Move the chicken to a container and reserve the chicken broth until ready to use.

2. Warm the coconut oil in a nonstick frying pan on moderate heat, then put in the onion and drizzle with Tex-Mex seasoning, salt, and pepper. sauté for five minutes until the onion is translucent.
3. Pour over the reserved chicken broth and coconut cream. Bring them to a simmer for about twenty minutes or until it becomes thick.
4. Put in the chicken, pumpkin seeds, paprika powder, lime juice, and cilantro to the soup. Stir to blend well before you serve.

Nutritional Info: calories: 730 ‖ total fat: 63g ‖ net carbs: 19g ‖ fiber: 9g ‖ protein: 23g

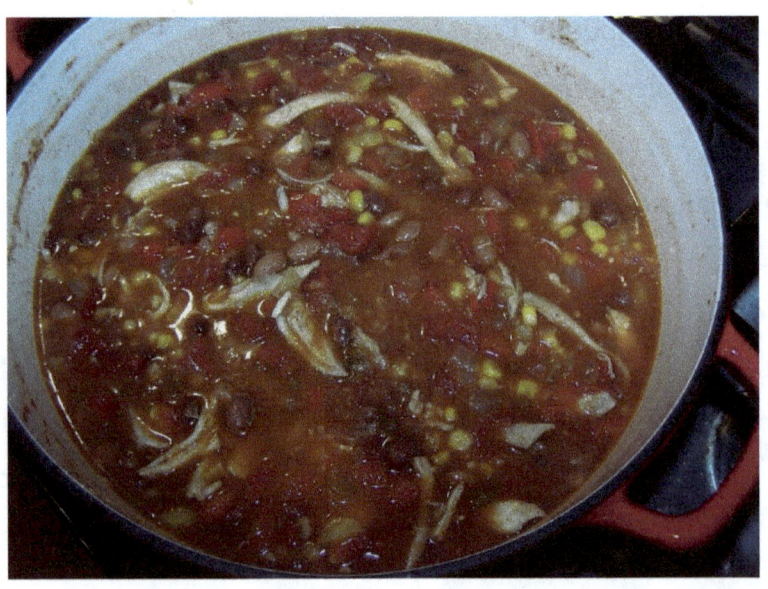

Thai Chicken Noodle Soup

Time To Prepare: ten minutes
Time to Cook: ten minutes
Yield: Servings 2-3

Ingredients:

- 6 cups low-sodium chicken broth
- 1 stalk lemongrass, minced
- 1 bay leaf
- 1 tablespoon ginger, grated
- 1 big carrot, cut
- 1 cup broccoli florets, trimmed
- 1 cup mushrooms, quartered
- ½ teaspoon. cayenne pepper
- 3 cloves garlic, minced
- 2 Tablespoon. gluten-free soy sauce
- Salt and black pepper (to taste)
- a handful of fresh cilantro, chopped
- 1-2 fresh chicken breasts, chopped
- 1/4 cup fresh lime juice
- 1/4 cup coconut milk
- 8-10 oz. gluten-free flat Thai rice noodles

Directions:
1. Boil noodles in accordance with package directions, or until firm to the bite. Drain and save for later.
2. Pour chicken broth in a big pot and bring to its boiling point using high heat. Put in chicken, broccoli, mushrooms, lemongrass, ginger, carrot, bay leaf. Turn heat to high and let the broth boil for a minute. Cover the pot and decrease the heat to moderate. Simmer the soup for 6 more minutes.
3. While the soup is simmering, mix in cayenne, garlic, lime juice, and soy sauce. Turn heat to low and put in the coconut milk; stir thoroughly.
4. Put cooked noodles into bowls. Pour soup over the noodles, then drizzle with cilantro.

Nutritional Info: Calories: 503 kcal ‖ Protein: 48.11 g ‖ Fat: 19.63 g ‖ Carbohydrates: 35.9 g

Thai Winter Vegetable Soup

Time To Prepare: 60 minutes
Time to Cook: 6 hours
Yield: Servings 12

Ingredients:

- ½ Of Lemon Juice
- 1 Lime Juice
- 1 Piece Ginger (Peeled, Grated)
- 1 Teaspoon Cumin
- 14 Ounce Coconut Milk
- 14 Ounce Peeled Italian Plum Tomatoes
- 2 Large Onions (Peeled, Quartered)
- 2 Stalks Lemongrass (Split)
- 3 Carrots (Peeled, Chopped)
- 3 Cloves Garlic (Peeled, Chopped)
- 3 Red Bell Peppers (Quartered, Seeded)
- 4 Large Sweet Potatoes (Peeled, Cut)
- 4 Tablespoons Cilantro (Chopped)
- Ground Black Pepper
- Optional: 1 Green Chili Pepper (Chopped)
- Salt

Directions:

1. Cook the vegetables with ginger and chili before pouring in coconut milk.
2. Mix in cilantro, cumin, lemon juice, and seasoning, cooking for around six hours.
3. Remove lemongrass and blend until thick.
4. Put in lime juice, seasoning, and cilantro to serve.

Nutritional Info: Calories: 468 kcal ‖ Carbohydrates: 81 g ‖ Fat: fifteen g ‖ Protein: 8.5 g

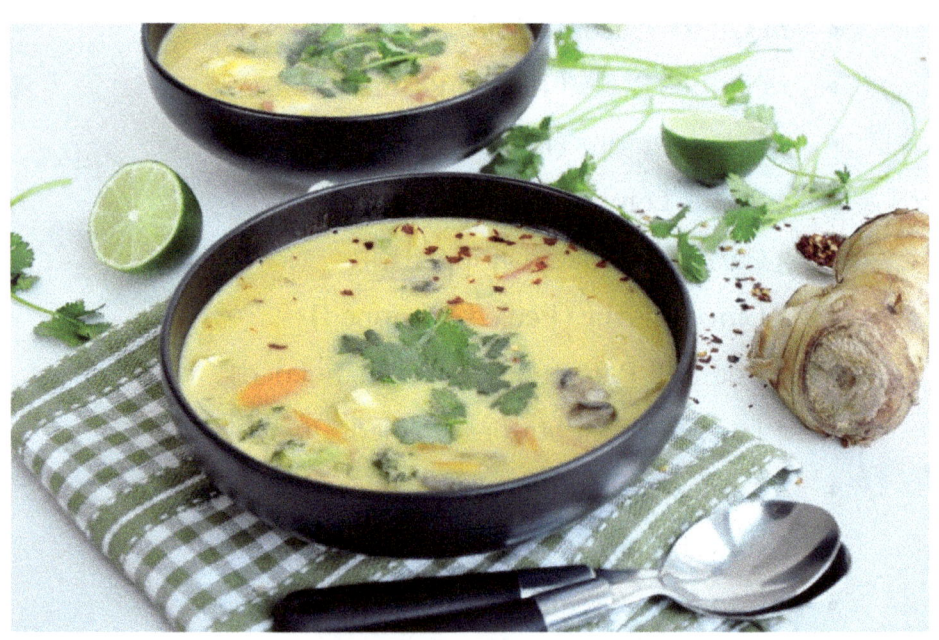

DESSERTS

Spiced Tea Pudding

Time To Prepare: ten minutes
Time to Cook: ten minutes
Yield: Servings 3

Ingredients:

- ½ cup coconut flakes
- ½ teaspoon cloves
- 1 ½ cups berries
- 1 can coconut milk
- 1 cup almond milk
- 1 tablespoon chia seeds
- 1 tablespoon ground cinnamon
- 1 tablespoon raw honey
- 1 teaspoon allspice
- 1 teaspoon cardamom
- 1 teaspoon green tea powder
- 1 teaspoon nutmeg
- 2 tablespoons pumpkin seeds
- 2 teaspoons ground ginger

Directions:

1. In your blender, puree tea powder with coconut milk, almond milk, cinnamon, coconut flakes, nutmeg, allspice, cloves, honey, cardamom, and ginger split into bowls. Heat a pan on moderate heat, put in berries until bubbling, then move to your blender and pulse well. Split the berries into the bowls with the coconut milk mix, top with chia seeds and pumpkin seeds before you serve.
2. Enjoy!

Nutritional Info: ‖ Calories: 150 ‖ Fat: 6 ‖ Fiber: 5 ‖ Carbohydrates: 14 ‖ Protein: 8

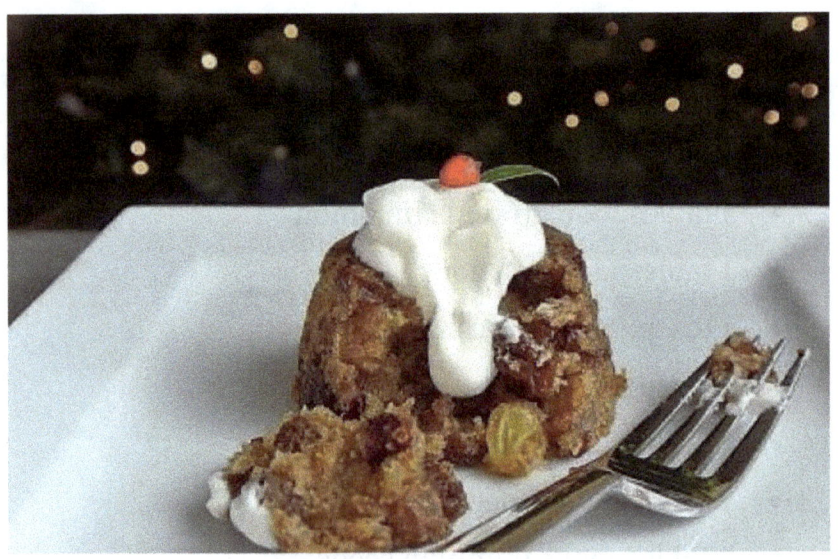

Spicy Popper Mug Cake

Time To Prepare: five minutes
Time to Cook: five minutes
Yield: Servings 2

Ingredients:

- ¼ teaspoon sunflower seeds
- ½ a jalapeno pepper
- ½ teaspoon baking powder
- 1 bacon, cooked and cut
- 1 big egg
- 1 tablespoon almond butter
- 1 tablespoon cashew cheese
- 1 tablespoon flaxseed meal
- 2 tablespoons almond flour

Directions:

1. Take a frying pan then place it on moderate heat
2. Put cut bacon and cook until they have a crunchy texture
3. Take a microwave proof container and mix all of the listed ingredients(including cooked bacon), clean the sides

4. Microwave for 75 seconds making to put your microwave to high power
5. Take out the cup and slam it against a surface to take the cake out
6. Decorate using a bit of jalapeno and serve!

Nutritional Info: ‖ Calories: 429 ‖ Fat: 38g ‖ Carbohydrates: 6g ‖ Protein: 16g

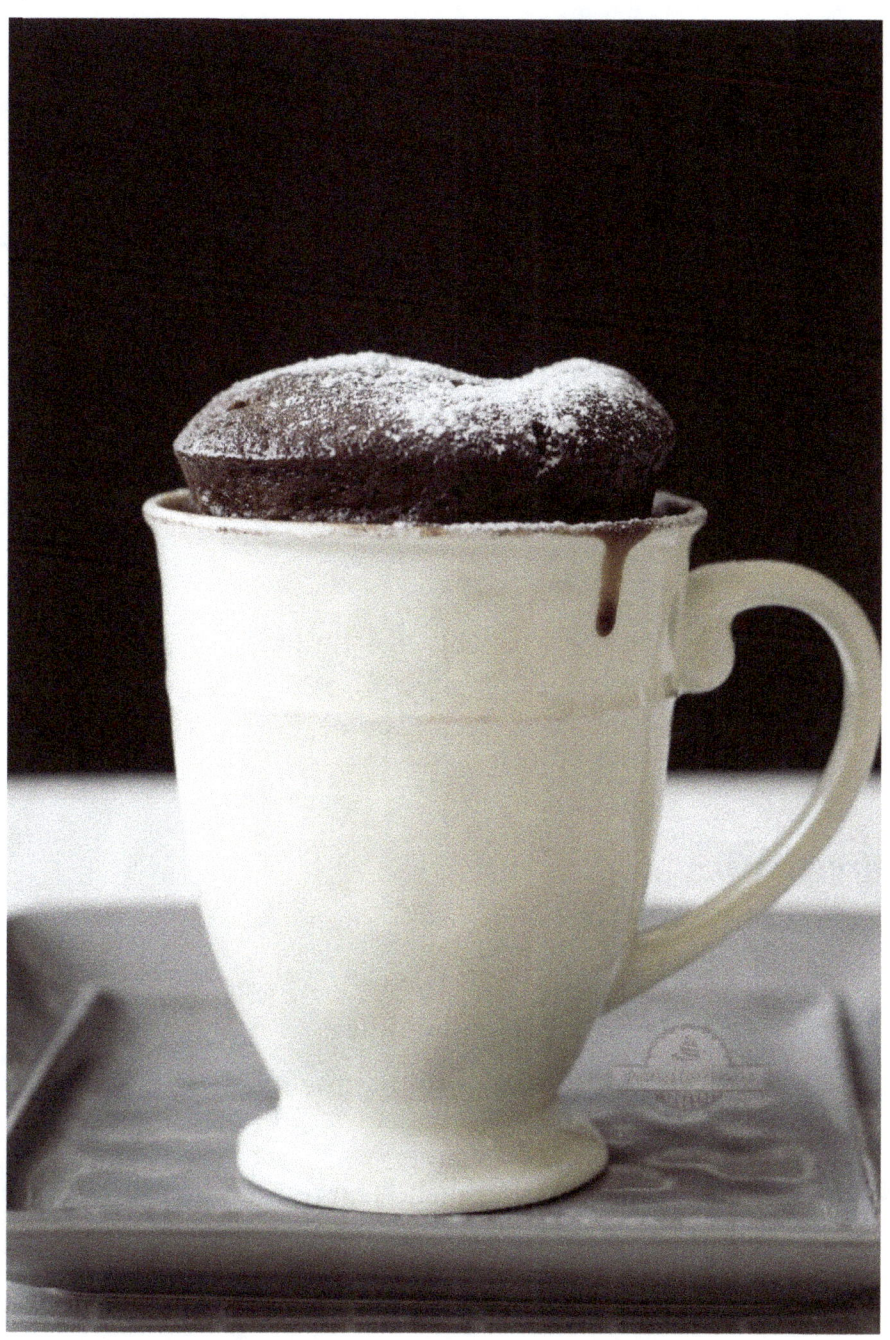

Strawberry Granita

Time To Prepare: ten minutes
Time to Cook: ten minutes
Yield: Servings 8

Ingredients:

- ¼ teaspoon balsamic vinegar
- ½ teaspoon lemon juice
- 1 cup of water
- 2 lb. strawberries, halved & hulled
- Agave to taste
- Just a small pinch of salt

Directions:

1. Wash the strawberries in water.
2. Keep in a blender. Put in water, agave, balsamic vinegar, salt, and lemon juice.
3. Pulse multiple times so that the mixture moves. Blend until smooth.
4. Pour into a baking dish. The puree must be 3/8 inch deep only.
5. Place in your fridge the dish uncovered till the edges start to freeze. The center must be slushy.

6. Stir crystals from the edges lightly into the center. Stir thoroughly to mix.
7. Chill till the granite is nearly fully frozen.
8. Scrape loose the crystals like before and mix.
9. Place in your fridge once more. Using a fork, stir 3-4 times till the granite has become light.

Nutritional Info: Calories 72 ‖ Carbohydrates: 17g ‖ Fat: 0g ‖ Sugar: 14g ‖ Fiber: 2g ‖ Protein: 1g

Strawberry Ice Cream

Time To Prepare: 5 Minutes
Time to Cook: 5 Minutes
Yield: Servings 2-3

Ingredients:

- 1 Banana, frozen & cut
- 1 cup Strawberries, frozen
- 1 tsp. Vanilla extract
- 2 tbsp. Coconut Milk

Directions:

1. Begin by placing strawberries and banana in a high-speed blender and blend it for two to three minutes.
2. While you blend, spoon in the coconut milk, and the vanilla extract.
3. Carry on blending until the mixture is thick and smooth.
4. Serve the ice-cream instantly since it does not keep well in the freezer.

Nutritional Info: ‖ Calories: 78 Kcal ‖ Protein: 1g ‖ Carbohydrates: 13.6g ‖ Fat:2.7g

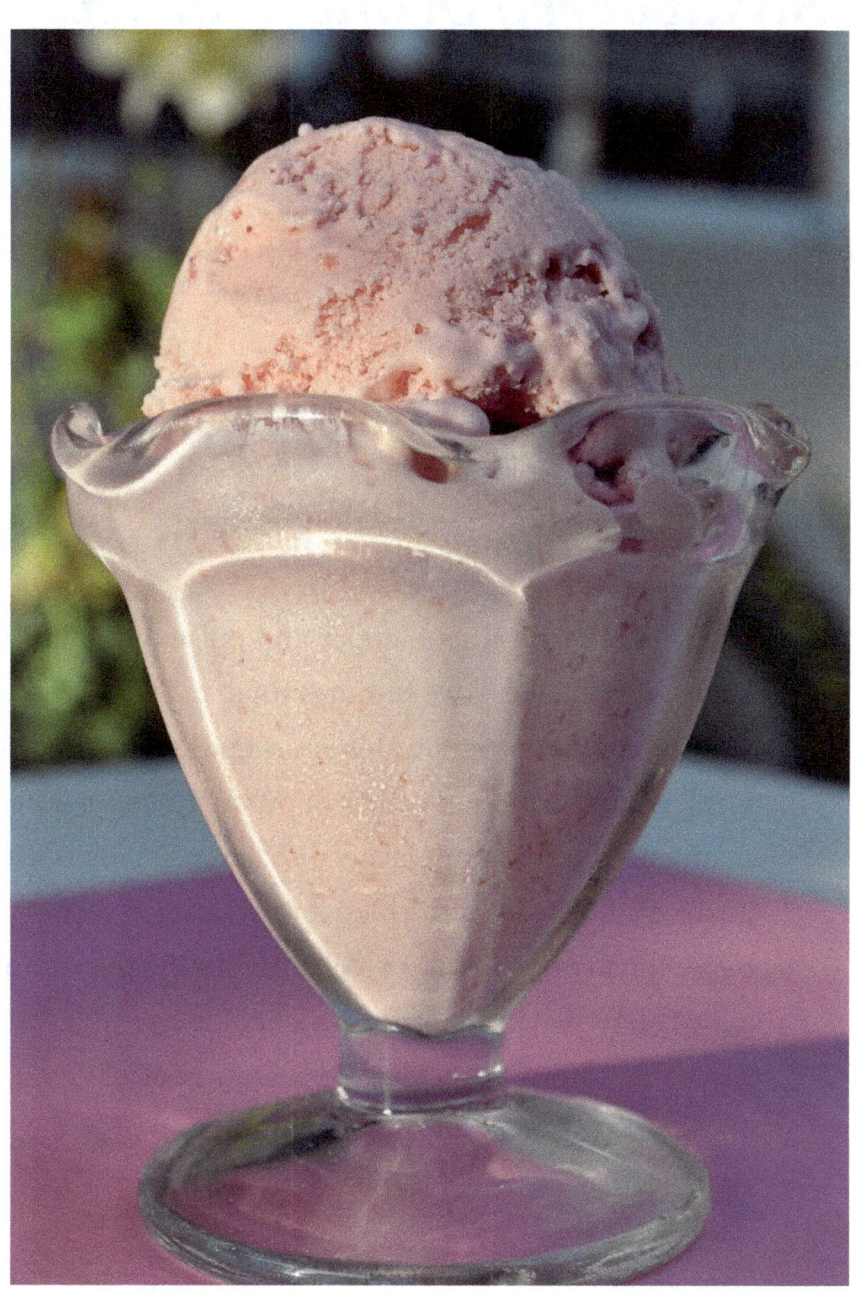

Strawberry Orange Sorbet

Time To Prepare: five minutes
Time to Cook: 0 minutes
Yield: Servings 3

Ingredients:
- 1 cup Orange juice or coconut water
- 1 pound Frozen strawberries

Direction:
1. Pour strawberries in a blender and pulse until all you have left are flakes. two minutes tops.
2. Now put in the coconut water or orange juice and pulse until you get a nice and smooth puree. Have a spatula handy because you might need to scrape some of the puree off the walls of the blender sometimes.
3. Serve the moment you're done or put in the freezer for about forty-five minutes for a sorbet feel.
4. Also, you can pour the smoothie into popsicle molds and freeze for hours or even overnight.
5. Enjoy!

Nutritional Info: ‖ Calories: 118 kcal ‖ Protein: 2.88 g ‖ Fat: 2.19 g ‖ Carbohydrates: 23.25 g

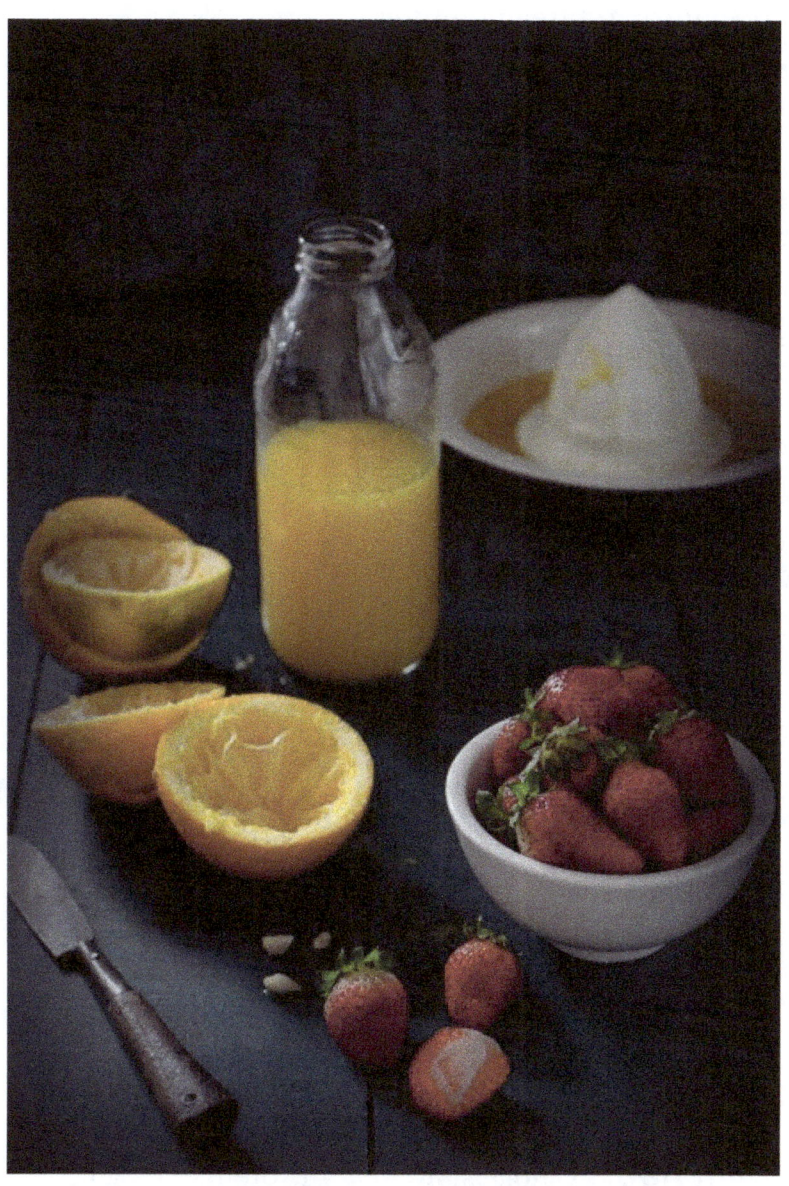

Strawberry Shortcake

Time To Prepare: fifteen minutes
Time to Cook: 0 minutes
Yield: Servings 4

Ingredients:

- .25 cup Semi-sweet chocolate chips
- 1 tbsp. Low-calorie margarine
- 12 hulled Strawberries
- 2.3-inch Shortcake, quartered

Directions:

1. Using waxed paper, line a cookie sheet.
2. Thread 2 shortcake pieces and 3 strawberries on 4 skewers.
3. In a small deep cooking pan, mix together the margarine and chocolate chips before placing the deep cooking pan on the stove over a burner turned to low heat. Stir until the ingredients are well mixed.
4. Sprinkle the chocolate onto the kabobs and then put them in your fridge for about four minutes to cool.

Nutritional Info: ‖ Calories: 40 kcal ‖ Protein: 1.85 g ‖ Fat: 2.3 g ‖ Carbohydrates: 3.32 g

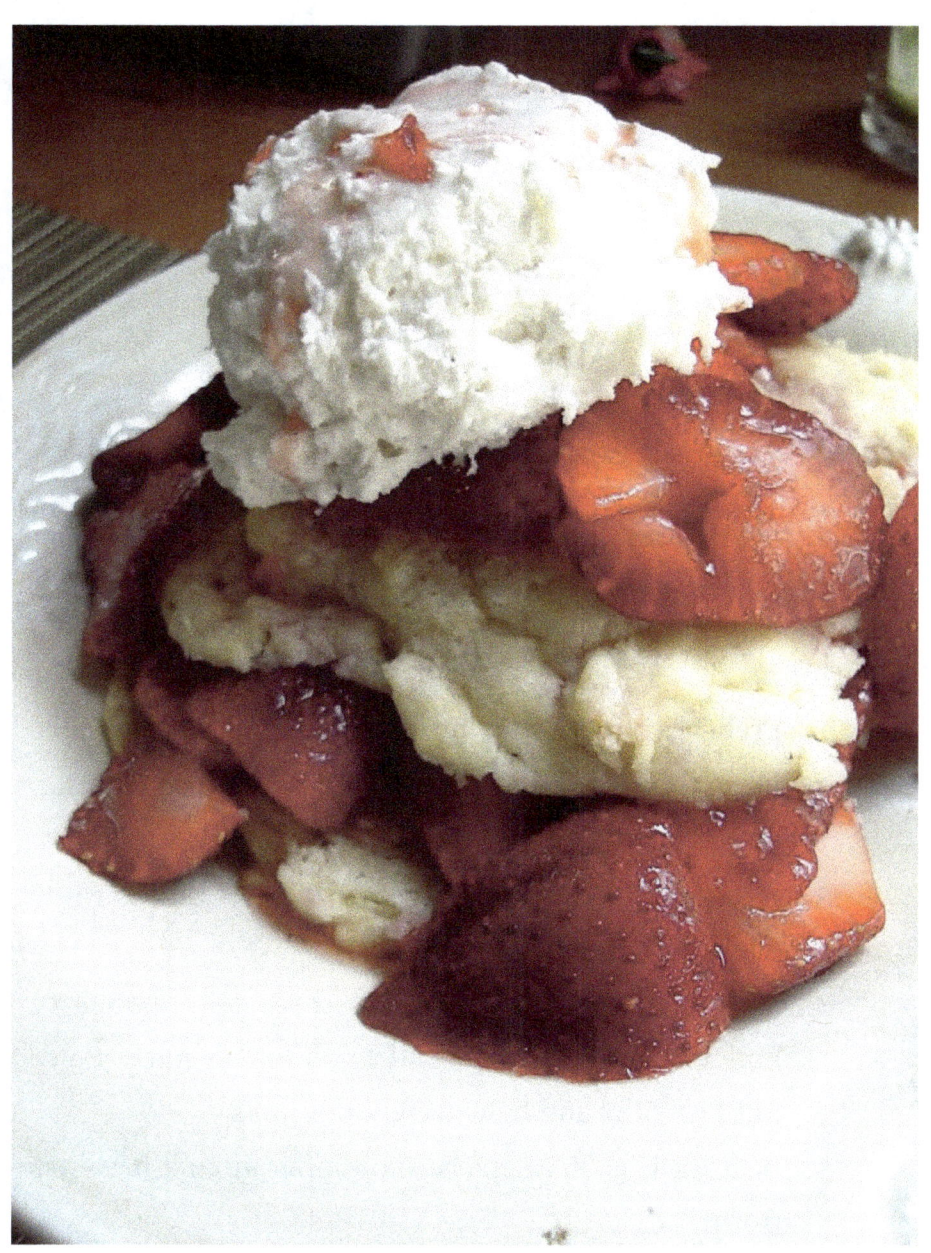

Strawberry Soufflé

Time To Prepare: fifteen minutes
Time to Cook: twelve minutes
Yield: Servings 6

Ingredients:

- 18 ounces of fresh strawberries, hulled
- 5 organic egg whites, divided
- 4 teaspoons of fresh lemon juice
- 1/3 cup of raw honey, divided

Directions:

1. Preheat your oven to 350F.
2. Place the strawberries in a blender then pulse until a puree form.
3. Strain the strawberry puree using a strainer while discarding the seeds.
4. Mix the strawberry puree to three tablespoons of honey, two egg whites, and fresh lemon juice. Pulse until a frothy and light-weight develops.
5. Beat the eggs in a separate container up to it becomes frothy.
6. Put in the remaining honey and beat until a stiff peak forms.

7. Gently- fold the egg whites into the strawberry mixture.
8. Move the mixture toto six big ramekins and place them on a baking sheet.
9. Bake for around 10-twelve minutes.
10. Take out of the oven and serve instantly.

Nutritional Info: ‖ Calories: 100 ‖ Fat: 0.3g ‖ Carbohydrates: 22.3g ‖ Sugar: 19.9g ‖ Protein: 3.7g ‖ Sodium: 30mg

Sweet Almond And Coconut Fat Bombs

Time To Prepare: ten minutes + twenty minutes chill time
Time to Cook: 0 minutes
Yield: Servings 4

Ingredients:

- ¼ cup melted coconut oil
- 3 tablespoons cocoa
- 9 and ½ tablespoons almond butter
- 9 tablespoons melted almond butter, sunflower seeds
- 90 drops liquid stevia

Directions:

1. Take a container and put in all of the listed ingredients
2. Combine them well
3. Pour scant 2 tablespoons of the mixture into as many muffin molds as you prefer
4. Chill for about twenty minutes and pop them out
5. Serve and enjoy!

Nutritional Info: ‖ Total Carbohydrates: 2g ‖ Fiber: 0g ‖ Protein: 2.53g ‖ Fat: 14g

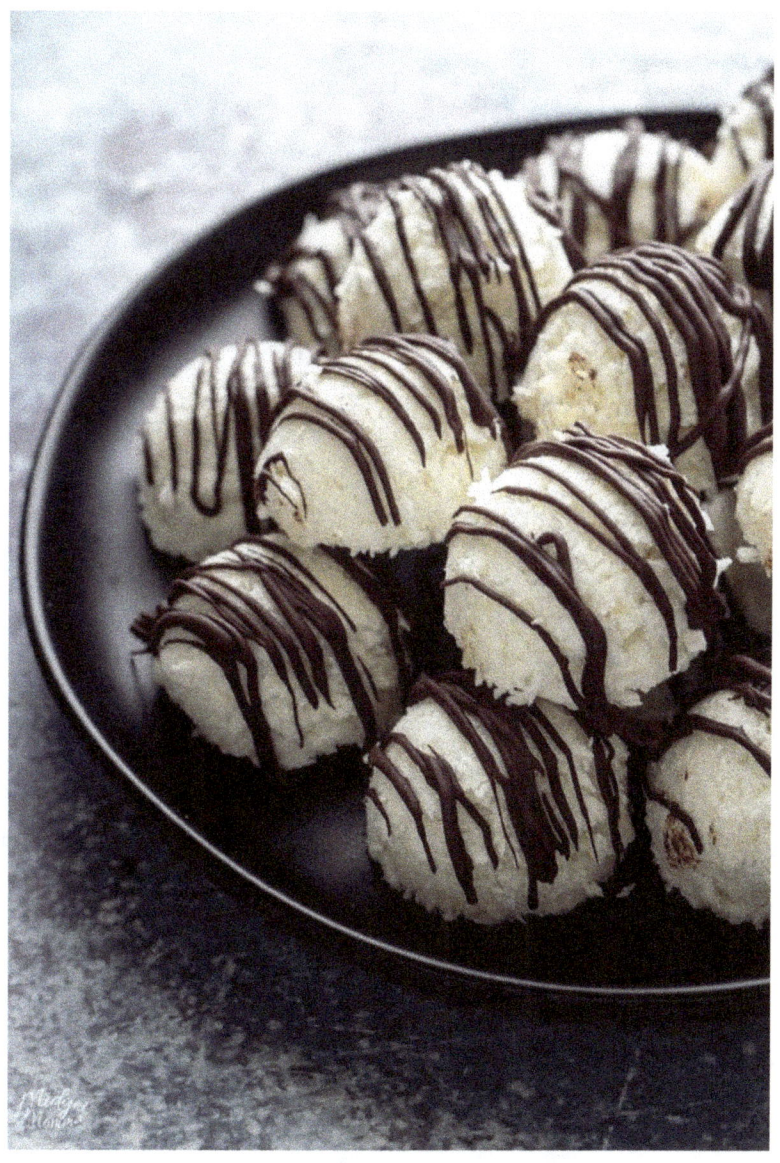

The Most Elegant Parsley Soufflé Ever

Time To Prepare: five minutes

Time to Cook: six minutes

Yield: Servings 5

Ingredients:

- 1 fresh red chili pepper, chopped
- 1 tablespoon fresh parsley, chopped
- 2 tablespoons coconut cream
- 2 whole eggs
- Sunflower seeds to taste

Directions:

1. Preheat the oven to 390 degrees F
2. Almond butter 2 soufflé dishes
3. Place the ingredients to a blender and mix thoroughly
4. Split batter into soufflé dishes and bake for about six minutes
5. Serve and enjoy!

Nutritional Info: ‖ Calories: 108 ‖ Fat: 9g ‖ Carbohydrates: 9g ‖ Protein: 6g

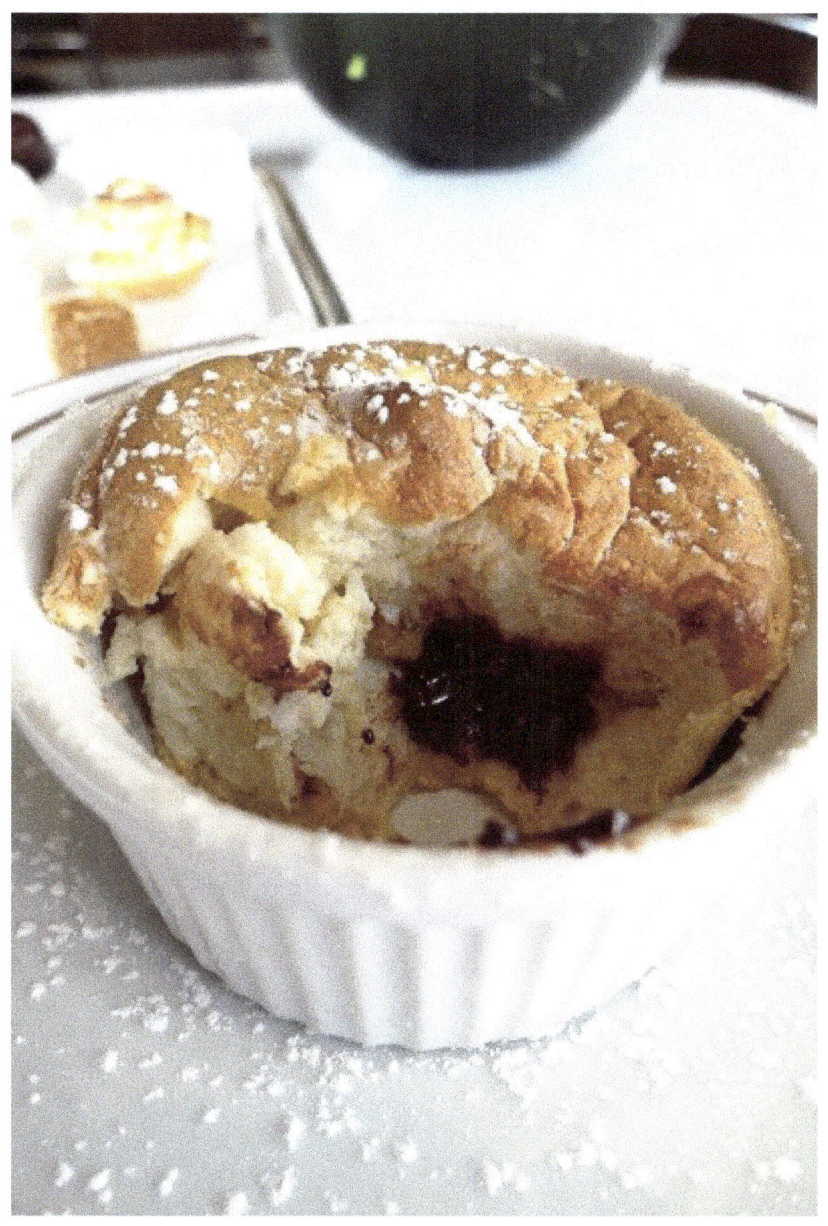